THE FINAL CHOICE

End of Life Suffering:
Is Assisted Dying the Answer?

CARALISE TRAYES

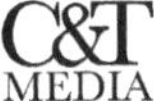

"The decision about whether or not to legalise euthanasia is the single most important values decision of the 21st century."
– Professor Margaret Somerville

"We are offering sanctuary and serenity, and a safe harbour where people can peacefully make their own choice. Opponents will do and say just about anything to undermine it."
– David Seymour MP

"It runs against every benefit of the law that protects human life that we have had in our country since the legal system was established."
– Grant Illingworth QC

"I am the doctor potentially injecting this lethal drug. I have to be for, or against. I can't abstain from this."
– Dr Sinéad Donnelly

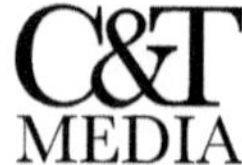

Capture & Tell Media
Email: contact@captureandtell.nz
www.captureandtell.nz

Front cover photography: Kevin Carden
Back cover photography: Twigs & Sticks Media
Proofreading: Mary Dobbyn
Typesetting and layout: Janet Curle

National Library of New Zealand (Te Puna Matauranga o Aotearoa)
Title: The Final Choice. End of Life Suffering: Is Assisted Dying the Answer?

ISBN: 978-0-473-52451-7 (pbk)
ISBN: 978-0-473-52452-4 (epub)

Subjects: Euthanasia, Assisted Dying, Medical / Nursing / Palliative Care, Social Science: Death & Dying, Family & Relationships: Death, Grief & Bereavement, Life Stages / Later Years, Medical / Nursing / Social, Ethical & Legal Issues, New Zealand Non-Fiction

First printing 2020 New Zealand
International listing 2020 www.ingramspark.com

CONTENTS

PREFACE

My mum said something profound to me the other day. She told me I'm part of a generation that for the first time in history has seen a global, unified response to an invisible threat.

Never in the history of humanity have more than 180 nations across the world closed their borders and put their nations into a coma to stem a pandemic like COVID-19. It's an unprecedented move of solidarity that will forever be marked in the books of mankind. A commonality that has spanned cultures, continents and civics like only a few other things in life can.

It's forced people on the front lines of the medical field to make impossible decisions over which lives are worth saving, and compelled nations to put the economy in second place to the health of its citizens. For many it's brought us face to face with the uncomfortable reality of death. Yet in the midst of isolation it has also forced us to consider how we live life.

It's a strange time then to be faced with another life-and-death dilemma when, during the same year, we will be confronted with a vote on an assisted dying law change in our elections in New Zealand.

Yet here we are.

It's an ever-stranger turn of events for me to be sitting in my converted home office interviewing people in their homes from across New Zealand, and the world, for this book that was only an idea a few months ago.

As with the start of any good adventure, it was a curiosity that sparked the search. And good friends.

I got a call to do a freelance writing job for a friend and as part of the task, I attended a meeting where assisted dying was discussed. In retrospect, I can see I was naive in my agreement to tag along thinking it would be an easy way to earn a bit of money for our 'nappy funds'. As a mum of two young children, even an outing that included talking about the legality of dying was a holiday.

The job finished, but it was then that something else began: I discovered the enormity and seriousness of the End of Life Choice Act us Kiwis will be voting on.

Like many of us, I thought the approaching vote was a simple 'yes' or 'no' tick box question around whether we would allow people the right to choose how and when they want to die. Even the fact that I knew there was a binding referendum has apparently put me ahead of a huge number of New Zealanders who don't know it's due to be connected with the elections in 2020.

But following that meeting, and as I began reading, I found myself with more questions than answers. What actually is assisted dying? Who wants to use it? Will it bring relief to people suffering, and if so, why is there resistance to it? Why are doctors and lawyers, ethicists and disabled people hitting headlines for and against it? And why are we voting about it in a binding referendum?

I also found high-ranking voices making claims that this is, "The biggest decision our generation will face", and that, "This law could change the fabric of society". Was this just scaremongering?

It's probably because of the journalistic sense of seeking out answers which is wired into my being after ten years in the field that makes it irresistible for me to follow a lead. Every time I hear sirens and see a fire engine my heart rate increases and my palms get sweaty. There were plenty of emergencies I chased down for newspaper headlines in my years reporting for Fairfax Media outlets, and my instincts still kick in.

So when an idea of following my questions and writing a book full of answers arose, it was hard to resist. If I have questions that need answering before I can in good conscience put my pen to a vote, then most other New Zealanders will too.

One thing I learnt while working in the community—people are the best resource, provide the greatest interest, and hold the most value. So it's people I pursue to pose questions to in the pages ahead.

I've chosen who to interview by sifting through the Justice Select Committee submissions received when the End of Life Choice Act was before Parliament. These are people who have enough vested interest to lodge their comment. Many have spoken out publicly in the media before.

From among them are specialists and ethicists, those who are terminally ill and positively well, passionate advocates and their opposites. Some are found within the fabric of our nation, and others carry experience from their own jurisdictions internationally.

What I discovered early on was that the common voice in favour of the law change was endearingly simplistic. So in many cases I presented this case before those in opposition.

Initially I assumed this issue would provoke some religious reaction around sanctity of life and 'playing God', but while interviewing I found religion often did not determine which side someone sat on. In fact, it was seldom relevant to anyone's reasoning. As one ethicist said, "This is not a religious issue, but a societal issue."

I recognise the topic may provoke a variety of feelings—death always does. My hope is that you will walk away from this book knowing more. Thinking more. Talking more about your future and the future of your loved ones. Being better equipped for compassion. Better informed about legislation. And maybe even being inspired to be a better person. To be a little less afraid to look at dying and be more free to live.

SECTION 1:

INTRODUCTION

Vicki Walsh and Lecretia Seales. Both New Zealanders were in their early 40s when they were diagnosed with brain cancer glioblastoma multiforme in the same year. Both women were highly committed to their work and were fiercely independent. Neither wanted to die. And both chose to fight the illness. Yet Lecretia succumbed and Vicki lived on.

Most of us Kiwis have heard or read Lecretia's story. It's been told through documentaries, features and blogs. In her final years, she dedicated herself to seeing the law change to allow for assisted dying—something she believed would bring relief not only to herself, but also to those that followed.

Lecretia's story has been instrumental in paving the way for the End of Life Choice Act (EOLC Act). It highlights the key arguments for the law change to provide a choice to end a life with medical assistance.

Vicki's story is a little more hidden. She didn't take a case against the High Court or get picked up by news agencies. You probably won't recognise her face or be familiar with her name. Yet her tale and stance are still as poignant and integral.

Lecretia is no longer here as an ambassador for assisted dying. But her mum, Shirley Seales, has taken up the cause, albeit cautiously.

Vicki is ready in waiting for my call in her living room in Palmerston North.

CHAPTER 1:

VICKI WALSH

"Personal Account

Vicki Walsh knew something wasn't right when she narrowly escaped a serious car crash while driving home one Friday night.

She had approached an intersection and went to put the brakes on… but her foot refused to cooperate. Panic slowed the scene before her eyes. Thankfully her other foot listened, slamming the brakes hard and saving her from an approaching car. The incident left her shaking, but Vicki took it as a sign she needed to rest.

The Palmerston North Department of Corrections prison manager and mum of two had been pushing herself hard at work and studying part time. She'd just finished a two-and-a-half-hour run with a friend.

But when Vicki returned to work on Monday things hadn't improved. "I was standing at my desk and all of a sudden I couldn't speak, I couldn't walk, and I had tears streaming down my face. It was like everything had frozen," Vicki says.

A knock eventually came at the door and something snapped inside Vicki, allowing her to regain control. "My husband, Dave, had come to visit me. He took one look at my face and he was frightened." From there the couple went straight to see a doctor.

Vicki had a seizure in the waiting room. Tests and an MRI were done. The doctor sat with Vicki and told her, "You've got a mass on your brain". In that moment her life was turned upside-down.

At 43 years old Vicki was diagnosed with glioblastoma multiforme (GBM), one of the most aggressive forms of cancer which starts in the brain. She was told she had 12 to 14 months to live. Incredibly, that was eight years ago.

The doctor sat with Vicki and told her, "You've got a mass on your brain". In that moment her life was turned upside-down.

There's no doubt Vicki Walsh is a cancer-fighting machine. The now-52-year-old grandmum has defied the odds—or in this case, the doctor's prognosis. She demonstrates life can be good, and long, despite terminal illness.

I've arranged to meet Vicki via a Messenger video call. She's sitting in a spare room in her 'jammies'. There's passion in her voice, despite her apology for being a bit croaky as she finished chemotherapy yesterday.

It's always a strange feeling knowing you are going to dive straight into the deep parts of someone's life story while barely knowing them.

We talk about having kids, Vicki's five grandchildren she's immensely proud of, and how much life changes when they come along... like how peeing alone in the toilet is no longer possible.

Vicki says being diagnosed with brain cancer was unbelievable. "I was fit, healthy, I exercised and ate well. I had a good paying job and had anything I wanted. But it was all taken in a moment."

Her husband, Dave, had to tell the kids, and she prepared for the intense surgery. "Everyone who came in to see me looked like someone had kicked them in the guts. It was a scary time."

Surgery wasn't smooth.

"I had a stroke during the operation. I had to learn how to use my leg again afterwards and I had chemotherapy and radiotherapy. It's hard to describe that time. It was such a blur. I went from 60kg to 99.9kg. Everything hurt."

Thankfully Vicki recovered well from the treatment and learned a new normal. There's been plenty of ups and downs through the process though. And she's glad assisted dying wasn't available during her dark moments.

"During the time this was all happening Brittany Maynard came to my attention. Her story was hitting the media in the United States and somehow it planted some seeds in my head that euthanasia and assisted dying was an honourable thing to do. Brittany also had GBM and wanted to have control of her life. I'm a control freak too so it started me thinking it's something I should consider."

In 2014, Brittany ended her life by assisted suicide. She was out walking her dog the morning before she did it.

"It made me feel gutless for not taking my life," Vicky says. "I never realised how strong subliminal messages really are."

One day at home Vicki considered her own suicide. "I knew there wasn't an easy way to lose someone you loved, so why not just go now? My kids were in a good place. I was loved by my husband. I didn't want them to have to go through a hard journey with me being sick, so in some ways it could be a blessing to die..."

"I didn't want them to have to go through a hard journey with me being sick, so in some ways it could be a blessing to die..."

She counted out enough pills to kill herself. But before she took them a thought crossed her mind, "Have a cup of tea first and think about it". It's amazing what a good cup of tea can do. During that time she had a change of heart. "What I didn't realise was that I was depressed."

If depression could knock at the door of someone with solid love and support from friends and family, it would surely be a threat to those with little or no support, Vicki says. "Giving someone the ability to make a life-and-death choice while they are influenced by depression is ridiculous. It's like handing out nooses in a suicide clinic."

If you'd asked Vicki before her accident if she thought assisted dying was a good idea, she would have said, "Yes, it's your right to choose".

"But now I realise that—yes, if you could go around with your head in a paper bag then it would be OK... but you can't. You live in a world with others. I don't want to see people in pain and suffering; I want people to get the palliative care they deserve."

Bringing dignity to dying is something those in favour of the law change are adamant it will achieve. But to Vicki it's the wrong way around.

"It's not about dying with dignity; it's about living with dignity. It's about how we treat people so they can live with dignity. To truly help someone is to ease their suffering by having the correct support in place—it's not simply thinking we can relieve someone by ending their life."

"It's not about dying with dignity; it's about living with dignity."

When Vicki was first diagnosed she was told she would live 12 to 14 months if she didn't get sick.

"I got a virus. I had a stroke. But here I am, more than eight years later, living life. Sure my life doesn't look the same as it used to; but I'm glad I'm here."

Her life testifies: "Doctors get it wrong."

But the battle against cancer wasn't over for Vicki. It returned in 2019. "This time I knew. I saw all the symptoms. I asked for an MRI in July and it came back clear but the symptoms got worse. A few months later I went for another scan and the oncologist confirmed it. I was told last time I wouldn't be able to receive any treatment if it came back. The doctor had explained to me that this kind of cancer is like a weed. They had sprayed Roundup on it, but it was still there and it would pop up again. So I thought 'this was it'."

The surgeon called to talk about treatment options. "That shocked us—he said there were risks but I could get surgery and treatment again as it had been so long since the last one. He explained all the risks and I was like, 'Hell yeah, let's do it'."

With GBM the stats show only a few make it to five years. Most die within 24 months of being diagnosed. A lot die within six months. "But I'm testament to say that isn't always accurate."

Vicki expected weeks in hospital and a slow recovery. "I came out of surgery at 6.30pm on a Tuesday night and within 48 hours I was home and felt better than I had in years. Who would have thought a person diagnosed in 2011 would still be alive now? I'm lucky, and a special case. But who knows—there could be someone else like me."

Even though Vicki is doing well she is still deemed terminal. "If I didn't take my medication I'd be dead by lunchtime tomorrow. People often say to me, 'You're a cancer warrior' but I don't see myself like that. I'm an average person fighting for those who can't fight for themselves.

"I've talked to supporters of euthanasia and they say, 'it's for the lonely'. They say they're scared, frightened... but not one of them quoted pain. Those are sh*tty reasons. Why don't we fix those problems? If you want to help someone with a terminal illness love them unconditionally, through good and bad days. Be there for them always."

Vicki says both her kids changed her soiled pants when she was in paralysis after surgery. "They did it in a way so I didn't feel embarrassed. It's a true testament of love when someone takes care of you at your most vulnerable moment. My son was 21 when he did that. He did it like it was the most normal thing in the world. I didn't lose dignity. I'd ask my children—are you embarrassed by me? I walk

"It's a true testament of love when someone takes care of you at your most vulnerable moment."

with my leg dragging and my hair is falling out. I told them I would wear a wig or hat if they wanted. But, you know, they turned around and said, 'Mum, we're proud of you. It's hard for you to walk and you do it.' I feel like I'm teaching my kids resilience, that you don't give up when something is hard. My grandson asked, 'Nanny, is your hair going to fall out more?' And I said, 'yes'. Then he asked, 'Can I have some of your hair?' It doesn't bother children. Why does it bother us adults?"

Part of the problem is we don't see death or talk about it, Vicki says. "When someone is dying family members come from everywhere and no one prepares them. We have so much in place to prepare someone for the start of life like midwives, and courses, and support—but we don't do anything about death. It's as special as birth."

"We have so much in place to prepare someone for the start of life like midwives, and courses, and support—but we don't do anything about death. It's as special as birth."

Vicki says she lives day by day. And while she can't plan far ahead, she's very excited her granddaughter is visiting from Perth for the first time ever in July. "It's about having little things to enjoy. This weekend I'm hoping to stain more of my fence. And I'll feel like I've achieved a lot if I can do that," Vicki says. "Life is good."

While making my son breakfast this morning I watched a video clip by an organisation called Voice of Hope. The clip was about a group of young adults who had struggled with mental health.

The organisation has invited their families to an event in the guise of a movie preview, but they had actually secretly recorded personalised messages of thanks from each patient to their supporters. These young adults powerfully recognised the people who had stood with them through their illness and their heavy and dark days.

With emotions raw, I realised this issue is not just about someone wanting a dignified end of life... This is about how we treat people. How we stand with people and how we fight for them.

A tender moment in my interview with Vicki came when she spoke of people who came from far and wide after hearing about her terminal diagnoses.

There were still traces of hurt in her voice when she spoke of how some people would visit her for an hour or two, some would come back the next week, and some a few months. But very few came and walked with her through the whole recovery. She felt most people came to placate themselves rather than to support her. The ones who stayed made a world of difference. They carried her when she couldn't go on.

While I found that hard to receive, because of course you visit those going through a difficult time, it really challenged me. Who am I standing with? Who am I calling in on and checking in with? Am I supporting those in the deep, dark, and lonely places?

It may be uncomfortable at times, but stories like Vicki's can have an impact on the way we see the world. If we let them.

CHAPTER 2:

LECRETIA SEALES

"Personal Account

The End-of-Life Choice Society of New Zealand is hosting a general meeting which is open to the public. It's a good opportunity to meet the group strongly advocating for a change in the law. I want to better understand who they are and why they support this Act. And even better, their guest speaker is Lecretia's mum, Shirley Seales.

Lecretia was one of New Zealand's leading advocates for assisted dying and her story has been extremely influential in forming public opinion on the issue.

The 42-year-old Wellington lawyer died from a brain tumour in June 2015. Before she died, Lecretia took a case against the High Court to contest her right to die with assistance from her doctor. Lecretia's story is compelling and her death, tragic.

Walking into the Mt Eden War Memorial Hall on a Saturday afternoon I'm met with the sound of orchestral music and a woman singing opera. Surely there's not a performance before the meeting? I obviously really don't know what to expect.

After a quick look around I spot a small card on a nearby staircase with a hand-scrawled message: "EOLC Society meeting upstairs". The main hall downstairs is being used by a theatre production company rehearsing—sigh of relief.

It's quiet and orderly in the correct room as I slip in and take a back row seat. I'm the youngest by at least a decade. Society president Mary Panko is introducing Shirley and takes a few questions before getting under way.

"It's surprising to me how many people I speak to who don't even know we are having a binding referendum on this… We've got our work cut out," Shirley says. Well that's something in common for both sides of the argument.

I hear several foreign accents in the group of around 40 as questions are being raised about how to respond to people opposed to assisted dying. "I've been speaking to a practising nurse at hospice," one woman says. "She says anybody in Lecretia's position can have palliative care. How do we answer this? How do we educate people that hospice is there for some, but we need to move forward on euthanasia?"

Shirley responds: "My husband and I heard a presentation from a guy in Belgium who was visiting Tauranga, and over there it is hospice that offers assisted dying. That seems to me a common-sense approach… and they say it is a privilege to help someone to die. I hate all the, 'You can't possibly allow this because we just need to spend the money on palliative care'. Lecretia was so afraid of losing her mind it [having access to assisted dying] would have brought so much comfort. She squeezed every ounce of living out of every day. It was great to have hospice there to help her at home. I'm grateful for that." But the woman seems unsatisfied. There doesn't seem to be a direct answer to her question.

> **"Lecretia was so afraid of losing her mind it [having access to euthanasia] would have brought so much comfort."**

Shirley is welcomed with applause and quickly sets out to share a bit of her own story before revealing details around Lecretia's discovery of a tumour and her journey to the end. "My father left us when I was 11 and decided to bring his mistress into the family home," she says. "So Mum and us kids were out on the street. Mum did her best but wasn't well and died when I was 15."

Shirley admits she is reading a speech she had prepared for a previous meeting, but is earnest and open as she shares.

"I got pregnant with Lecretia when I was 16. I married her father Larry, who is here with me today. Lecretia felt she always owed me—that I had given up my life for her and my younger years, which was inaccurate. She didn't get me pregnant and what's more, she was the best thing that ever happened to us. At least with Lecretia dying it gave us time to talk. Lecretia was not only my eldest daughter, but my best friend. I miss her terribly. One of the hardest things as a parent is watching a child die and not being able to fix it."

Before Lecretia was diagnosed she was suffering from poor vision and pain. A visit to the optometrist and doctor only resulted in being told she was overworked and having migraines. "I was angry at the optometrist and doctor. But Lecretia was only disappointed in herself for allowing herself to be fobbed off when she knew it was serious," Shirley says.

After pushing for a scan a specialist told her what she suspected: a tumour on her brain. "While it was not possible to remove the tumour, she was advised that it was already pushing on her spinal cord, and if she did not have surgery immediately there was a likelihood she would go into a coma and die within weeks."

Lecretia could have chosen to refuse treatment and the outcome would have been a reasonably swift death, Shirley says. It was something she considered as the thought of a tumour eating away at her brain was "intolerable". "Being in control was so important to Lecretia. Had this law [EOLC Act] been current at the time she was diagnosed she wouldn't have needed to consider refusing treatment. She would have had the comfort of knowing this was not her last chance to have control over her death."

Her family begged her to give it a fighting chance, and so Lecretia agreed to surgery. "The operation was very dangerous and could have left her paralysed, blind, or dead. She remained very staunch as she didn't want any of us to worry.

"After her surgery Lecretia endured six-and-a-half weeks of radiation, which left her head severely burnt and caused her to lose her short-term memory. The treatment did not cure her but bought her extra time and relieved some of that excruciating pain."

"She felt she could make an impact as she was a well-respected lawyer who had a terminal illness."

Lecretia compared the pain of illness to not being able to have children, a major life disappointment. Before getting sick she'd tried for years to have a child but was unsuccessful, Shirley says. "She managed to get pregnant twice as a result of six rounds of IVF only to miscarry as late as 11 weeks. Not long before she died Lecretia had a conversation with her fertility specialist who sympathised with her for having a terminal illness. She told him having a terminal illness was not as difficult as not being able to have children."

In the four years between her diagnosis and death, despite major difficulties including increasing immobility and low immunity, Lecretia travelled to Argentina and Morocco with her husband and parents.

During her career Lecretia was dedicated to law reform and worked with the Law Commission. She was a private person but she chose to put her face to a campaign to change the assisted dying law. "She felt she could make an impact as she was a well-respected lawyer who had a terminal illness," Shirley says.

It started with an interview with *The Listener* and went on to her being interviewed by *Radio NZ* and *60 Minutes*. Then, writing to the Justice Minister, Lecretia asked if the Law Commission would investigate the issue of assisted dying. "She felt that the Law Commission was the best place for the investigation and she trusted the Commission to review the issue on a completely evidential basis – not afraid to present conclusions that might be controversial."

The request was denied, so Lecretia decided to take a human rights case against the Government to challenge her right to die.

"Lecretia was on huge doses of steroids to attempt to alleviate the increasing swelling of the tumour. She had lost her mobility and almost all of her sight. She was sleeping most of the time but somehow she summoned the strength to make it to court for most of the first day and the last part of the final day."

A pause from Shirley, and her tone and rhythm that had become heavy returns to a lighter direction.

"Lecretia was never afraid of dying. She believed in God and always helped others. She was aware, in the case of the brain tumour, she would experience pain that could not be controlled by medication. She did not wish to be so heavily sedated that she would be unaware of her surroundings or her loved ones; as far as she was concerned, that was not living but rather existing."

It was clear Lecretia was a strong and determined woman.

"She loved life and she squeezed as much as she possibly could out of every day. She never complained of how difficult life was for her. I do remember the day that she became so rigid we couldn't get her out of bed. The hospice nurse decided there was no choice but to insert a catheter. Lecretia never said a word but she looked at me with such an anguished look at the indignity of having this done."

"She loved life and she squeezed as much as she possibly could out of every day. She never complained of how difficult life was for her."

Shirley believes Lecretia would not have chosen to use assisted dying if it was an option, but having the choice would have brought comfort. Lecretia was well taken care of in her last few weeks with a hospital bed, carers visiting, and access to medication and support.

> **"Life is not always fair. While hers was cut short she achieved more than most do in a full life."**

On 5 June, 2015 Lecretia died surrounded by her husband and parents at home.

"Life is not always fair. While hers was cut short she achieved more than most do in a full life," Shirley says.

Shirley finishes to appreciative applause.

After a few moments digesting the emotional intensity of Shirley's story, Mary encourages members to join her at a market day on Waiheke Island handing out flyers and speaking with people. "We have bumper stickers being printed too."

In a surprise turn of events there's a rattle at the door; Act Party leader David Seymour MP slips into the back and pulls up a seat next to me. David is the author of the EOLC Act and an advocate for it at its highest level. He's spotted from the front and there's a hum of excitement at his presence. He's invited up front.

This is my first encounter with the political magician at work in the flesh. It's a worthy introduction to a man who has catapulted the issue into the political process and continued to push the plough into its current position. I love observing how the masters of politics weave their words and pack their punches in such edible packets of charm.

David thanked the group for 'sticking' with the cause and encouraged them to go ahead with their idea to get bumper stickers printed for their cars. "Don't worry about putting a sticker on your car—I have my face and name plastered over mine and it never gets damaged," he says. Everyone laughs.

In this environment David comes across a lot more natural. Obviously it's an easier audience and he doesn't have the media staring him down.

"We are committed to changing the law, and we have—it's on the statute book. The difficulty is the wee clause we had to put in to get the votes that says we have to pass the referendum."

Act Party polls on the issue conducted weekly since November 2019 show 58 per cent in favour, 24 per cent against and 20 per cent undecided. "We are much closer than we think. I want to tell you this so all of us are 100 per cent committed to winning."

He uses Brexit as an example of potential similarities. Polls showed 70 per cent in favour and 30 per cent against until it came down to a vote. In the end they scraped over the line with 51.9 per cent in favour of leaving the European Union. "The Brexit campaign got fixated on the idea that Turkey could join the EU and there are 180 million Turks that could come to the UK. Now you can say what you like about the prejudices that drive that thinking, but once they focused people's minds on that fact, they couldn't get past it. No doubt our opponents to the EOLC Act will be looking for those kinds of objections."

A warning followed concerning elections, campaigns and goalposts moving because of the COVID-19 pandemic. "It might be good for us, as it will make it more difficult for opponents to shift public opinion. People will worry about something else, so they will just go with their default vote."

Summing up, David invokes confidence. "We have a number of

"We have a number of advantages. First of all, I'm right and they're wrong," David Seymour says.

"This is what could happen... but we are offering sanctuary and serenity and a safe harbour where people can peacefully make their own choice. Away from that horrible outcome," David Seymour says.

advantages. First of all, I'm right and they're wrong." Everyone claps.

"It's true: we have all the evidence on our side, and all the rubbish on the other. Eighty-eight per cent of Dutch still support their law 15 years on. So either the Dutch are more crazy that we realise or all the crap you hear is not true. We are morally right. People want a place of reassurance and serenity when they are at a difficult point in their life. That's what we offer. The other side is offering fear, uncertainty and doubt."

The troops have been rallied.

David says one of the strengths the Society has is their stories of people dying badly. "The public need to be reminded of that. This is what could happen... but we are offering sanctuary and serenity and a safe harbour where people can peacefully make their own choice. Away from that horrible outcome."

I have to acknowledge there's been an underlying tension in the history of journalism between politicians and reporters. And while I'm not wearing a journalist's hat these days I still have an instinctual caution around them.

There's something about the way David refers to the "serenity and safety" of a harbour that reminds me of a scene out of the Cameron Diaz and Tom Cruise film *Knight and Day*. In the film Cruise's character tells Diaz' to look out for keywords that indicate danger...

"They'll probably identify themselves as federal agents, and they'll DIP you."

"Dip me? In what?"

"Disinformation Protocol. They'll tell you a story about me, about how I am mentally unstable, paranoid... I'm violent and dangerous and it'll all sound very convincing."

"I am already convinced."

"Here's a few common DIP cue words to listen for: Reassuring words. Words like stabilised, secure, safe… If they say these words particularly with repetition, it means they're going to kill you."

"Oh, God!"

I realise I'm going to need to know a lot more about what the EOLC Act is and how we got here.

SECTION 2:

THE OVERVIEW

Before wading into an upcoming heated debate I need to gird myself with a bit of knowledge. How does this End of Life Choice Act actually work? Where did it come from and how did it get through the political process to a binding referendum?

I'm going to run through the basics of the Act and its process before dunking myself in opposite ends of the spectrum—by interviewing Euthanasia-Free New Zealand and the End-of-Life Choice Society representatives. I know they will provide a basic understanding of both camps. They will also introduce me to a variety of concepts and discussion around the issues which I will have to explore further.

Let's get going.

CHAPTER 3:

THE END OF LIFE CHOICE ACT

According to David Seymour, the purpose of the End of Life Choice Act is to give people with terminal illness the option of requesting assisted dying. "The Act includes provisions to ensure they are legally eligible and capable of making the decision of their own free will. And sets out a process in which it is done," he says.

So how would it actually work?

There are requirements around who is eligible for this. The person must be over 18 years old and be a New Zealand citizen or permanent resident. They must suffer from a terminal illness that will likely end their life within six months and experience unbearable suffering that cannot be relieved in a manner that they consider tolerable. They must have the ability to understand the nature and consequences of assisted dying and be deemed competent to make the decision.

It all starts when a person asks their doctor for assisted dying. That doctor then has a number of requirements to take the person through. They must provide the person with a prognosis on their condition and talk to them about the irreversible nature and anticipated impacts of assisted dying. They must also encourage the person to talk to family, friends and counsellors.

A doctor must do their best to ensure a person has not been pressured into the decision. And throughout the process they must also let the person know they can change their minds at any time. An application form is then filled in by both the doctor and the person (or someone on the person's behalf at their request if they cannot sign it themselves). A doctor can conscientiously object to being involved in this process but must refer the person on to a governing body.

Side note—there are three governing bodies to be established:

1) The SCENZ Group will be made up of nominated people to write standards of care, provide advice on medical and legal procedures, and offer practical assistance if requested. They will form a list of medical practitioners, psychiatrists and pharmacists willing to participate in assisted dying.

2) The registrar will be a nominated person who will maintain a register of forms lodged by applicants, co-sign prescriptions, establish procedures to deal with complaints, and report to the Minister of Health and an End of Life Review Committee.

3) The End of Life Review Committee's job is to consider the assisted death reports and recommend follow-up actions if it wasn't satisfied with those reports.

The signed form will be sent to the registrar and SCENZ Group. The Group will supply a second medical practitioner, who will examine the person and their files. They will fill in another form and send it to the registrar if they are satisfied by their findings.

If either of the doctors are uncertain of the person's competence they must jointly refer them to a specialist in mental health. The specialist must read the person's files, examine them, and give an opinion on whether they are competent, as well as fill in another form.

The application process is complete. Now the person waits to hear if they've been successful. If they are denied, they must be given a reason. If the application is granted, the person can now make arrangements with the medical practitioner around which option they would prefer: euthanasia or assisted suicide. And they are to choose a suitable time. When this time is chosen, the doctor needs to inform the registrar, who would check that forms have been filled in correctly. They must be notified at least 48 hours before administration.

The day arrives and the medical practitioner is ready to administer. The person must agree they want to receive the medication just before it is given. It's administered and the person dies. The death must be reported within 14 days to the registrar.

The Act itself is to be reviewed three years after its introduction with a report presented to Parliament, and every five years thereafter.

Sounds straight forward, right? Then why the controversy?

Previous attempts to legalise euthanasia

I hadn't realised this isn't the first rodeo for assisted dying bills in New Zealand. The issue had in fact been debated twice before in Parliament—once in 1995 with Michael Laws' Death with Dignity Bill, and a second in 2004 with Peter Brown's Death with Dignity Bill.

Then in 2015, a petition of nearly 9,000 signatures was headed by former Labour MP Maryan Street and made it to the steps of Parliament. That was around the same time Lecretia Seales' case was before the High Court.

The Government responded by sending it to the Health Select Committee to investigate public attitudes towards legislation permitting medically assisted dying. The committee received 21,000 submissions and the report released in 2017 stated it was clearly a very complicated, divisive and extremely contentious issue.

Maryan had drafted a bill but it was withdrawn as the Labour Party was busy in the lead-up to the then forthcoming election. That bill provided a road map for what we have today.

How did this Act get to referendum

Maryan Street wouldn't have been disappointed to see the End of Life Choice Bill plucked out of a biscuit tin in Parliament at around the same time her bill was denied. And yes, out of a biscuit tin. The blue-and-white tin itself is part of a 30-year parliamentary tradition, but it works essentially as a ballot box.

Any member of Parliament who isn't a minister can propose a law change by putting it on the ballot list. This gives MPs outside of government a chance to change policy with the random nature of the draw keeping it impartial. And that's how David Seymour's bill got its chance.

Every second Wednesday that Parliament sits, time is dedicated to debate these particular laws. When one bill has reached its conclusion, another one is drawn. Each bill that's pulled from the tin gets read in front of Parliament. This is called a 'first reading'. The MP in charge of the bill will introduce it, explain what's in it and say why they care about it.

In his introductory speech, David made a case that Kiwis should have this piece of legislation for democratic, legal and moral reasons. He said, "Seventy-five percent of New Zealanders who watched their loved ones die, often badly, feel they need more choice and control." That's the democratic reason.

The legal reason was highlighted in the case Lecretia Seales took to the High Court. The court basically ruled it was not at liberty to change the law—that was something the Government needed to do.

According to David, the most important reason by far is a moral one; for those who die in pain and suffering who can't be helped by palliative care.

As part of the first reading, MPs are welcome to make initial speeches. In all readings the Speaker of the House chooses some in favour and some opposed.

The EOLC Bill was to be a conscience vote, which means MPs could vote according to their own personal conscience, and on behalf of those they represent rather than to an official line set down by their political party.

MPs voted and the bill passed first reading on 13 December, 2017 with 76 MP votes in favour and 44 opposed.

Once passed, the bill was sent to a select committee. This one was sent to the Justice Select Committee. The public were invited to provide feedback through both written and oral submissions.

A select committee is made up of a selection of MPs and clerks, and between them they have the job to read and listen to all submissions and write a report which is to be sent back to Parliament. Often the report includes recommended changes. In a record-breaking response, 39,159 submissions were received on the EOLC Bill. Then followed 1,350 oral submissions being heard. That's a massive response and a huge workload.

A total of 114 SOPs was presented. Only three passed through voting.

Committee members hosted more than 40 public hearings in cities and towns across the country. It took 16 months before the committee got back to Parliament in April 2019. The final committee report only included limited recommendations to the Bill. This meant the weight of the work was put back on the shoulders of MPs in Parliament; something that some MPs said was a "failure to the process".

Why did the committee not produce significant recommendations? There was a fair amount of controversy surrounding the committee with complaints of tensions between MPs within the group. The report stated that the eight members on the committee held diverse views, and on many of the substantial issues "we did not decide".

The select committee report was tabled by Parliament. And the second reading began.

After a second vote 70 were in favour, 50 opposed. The margin of difference had decreased.

This brought the process to the Committee of the Whole House stage in July 2019. At this stage Parliament becomes a sort of select committee itself. Any MP can amend the bill being presented by submitting a Supplementary Order Paper (SOP). MPs debate on the SOPs then vote on them one by one. A total of 114 SOPs was presented.

Only three passed through voting—one of those was proposed by David Seymour, which was a pretty extensive rewrite of the Bill. His, among other things, narrowed the eligibility to those who are terminally ill with less than six months to live and ensured patients were the ones to initiate the assisted dying application process. That change was made explicitly to gain Green Party member votes. The second and third SOPs that passed added a requirement for a binding referendum, which ensured NZ First MPs would vote in support.

But that was contentious and divisive. Visible frustration came from some MPs—like Labour's Louisa Wall, who supports assisted dying but totally opposed it becoming a "public vote". "That is appalling and that is abhorrent," Louisa said. "You're putting us all in an untenable situation. My principles will not let me vote for the referendum—even if it means the bill fails."

"You're putting us all in an untenable situation. My principles will not let me vote for the referendum—even if it means the bill fails," says Louisa Wall.

Others, like National MP Alfred Ngaro, called it "irresponsible". "If in your hearts you know that this Bill is not safe enough, do not unleash this onto our country and into our nation where it will... do harm to our communities."

Labour's Willie Jackson told the House it was the "hardest vote" he'd ever had to make. "Referendums don't treat minorities well ... At the same time, I don't want to be the one vote that stops it all," he said.

All other SOPs were rejected. This issue was supposed to be a conscience vote, yet it's clear party play was still involved. Hello politics.

By 13 November, 2019 the Bill had its third and final reading and passed with 69 in favour and 51 opposed. The Bill became an Act.

Research in 2017 and 2019 revealed that while the majority supported assisted dying, many did not even know what it is, or in fact what it is not.

Referendum manoeuvre

Now usually the act would go straight to royal ascent where the Governor-General signs it in on behalf of the Queen. But for this Act to become operational it will have to have a majority vote in favour in the binding referendum which will be included in the 2020 General Elections. This is a highly unusual circumstance. Binding referendums to approve a specific law are just not done.

Those who support the referendum move say most Kiwis have been reading and are up with the play: they will make informed decisions when the time comes. After my research I would like to think I am going to make a sound decision.

But some other polling released by Curia Market Research has got me wondering. Research in 2017 and 2019 revealed that while the majority supported assisted dying, many did not even know what it is, or in fact what it is not. Results showed 74 per cent thought the Act would make it legal to turn off life support, and 70 per cent thought it would legalise the choice not to be resuscitated. These are both already legal. Of those surveyed 75 per cent think the EOLC Act would make euthanasia available to terminally-ill people only as a last resort, after all treatments have been tried to control their pain. This is not true. There were many other misunderstandings revealed.

If the EOLC Act passes the referendum with a majority of votes in favour, it becomes law. The fate of the Act now rests in the hands of us voting Kiwis.

> **Results showed 74 per cent thought the Act would make it legal to turn off life support, and 70 per cent thought it would legalise the choice not to be resuscitated. These are both already legal.**

"Do you support medical assistance to die for those experiencing irreversible, unbearable suffering at end-stage terminal disease?" I ask myself the poll question. A picture flashes into my mind...

It's the scene out of a war story. I'm sitting on the ground in the middle of a combat scene. There's chaos all around, the sounds of gunfire, men yelling, combat vehicles crashing through bush, smoke and fire are on the close horizon. A soldier kitted in full combat gear who has obviously just come off the front line has thrown himself in my arms—clinging to me in anguish. There is fear in his eyes, pain on his face. Dirt and sweat indicate signs of struggle.

I look down and he is severely injured. He cries out in pain. He is helpless. He is alone. "Please shoot me. Help me... shoot me."

The soldier is a victim, undeserving of the wounds received. My heart hurts for him. He looks in a bad way and I don't know if he will make it.

Should I take my gun and kill him? Is it compassionate to give him what he asks for? Or do I pick him up and carry him to the barracks? Back to safety and medical help, even if he might not survive. Would it be dignified for the soldier to die at the end of my gun? Or rather in the care and covering of his fellow countrymen, being carried through his last moments in the arms of one who is willing?

Justice Select Committee report summary

The Justice Select Committee met the thousands of New Zealanders who will directly be impacted by this law, passionate individuals both in favour and against it. I've looked for reviews on the submissions to gain a more ground-level impression of what was discovered and get a good basic lay of the land for my journey ahead.

The two best sources I came across was a Care Alliance review and a story by Stuff reporters Thomas Manch and Ruby Macandrew.

The Care Alliance report scrupulously analysed the submissions and found 91.8 per cent opposed the Bill. Similarly, 93.5 per cent of medical practitioners who had contributed were against it. Many submissions talked about a number of inadequacies around the safeguards in the Bill, but ultimately they concluded doctors ending the lives of patients far outweighs any benefits, the report said.

The Stuff report also agreed the "slippery slope" was a primary fear to many—"that the Bill would irrevocably change the country's view of death and would further loosen it in the future." Concerns came from the disability community that they would be unwillingly captured by a law that viewed their quality of life as lesser, the report said.

The Care Alliance report scrupulously analysed the submissions and found 91.8 per cent opposed the Bill.

Less than 10 per cent of submitters were in favour of the Bill.

Central arguments were that people should be given access to assisted dying on compassionate grounds. "In some instances they added the opinion that 'dignity in dying' could only be achieved by such means," the Care Alliance report said.

Both sides offered evidence from overseas jurisdictions which have legalised it, to bolster claims that such laws are safe, or conversely that they lead to people being killed without consent.

Statistical data is a funny thing. Interpretation can often be swung both ways. In one way I appreciate how such report's categorise submissions, tally feedback, and produce quantitative data. Yet I can't help but feel the true emotion, the personal stories, the expertise of opinion and the qualitative substance are lost in such practices. I want to hear who has spoken out. Why are the camps so vehemently and diametrically opposed? Why is the international data feeding into both sides?

While the majority of submitters to the committee opposed the Bill, a variety of polls have shown that New Zealanders are generally in support of assisted dying. Poll results show those in favour usually make up 58 to 74 per cent of respondents.

One Horizon poll surveying 1,300 people in April 2019 showed 74 per cent of adults supported medical assistance to die for those experiencing irreversible unbearable suffering at end-stage terminal disease, with 19 per cent opposed. Even if the person suffering wasn't facing immediate death, 65 per cent supported it.

My starting point for research and contacts is found within the pages of the committee submissions. I want to hear from medical specialists, those directly affected, and from people who understand how this law actually works. From people who are passionate and informed.

We are, after all, voting on an actual piece of law, not just on the concept of assisted dying.

Already taking shape is an emotional journey into some deep questions around the essence of life. I can't avoid it and I won't apologise for it—because it is needed; there are people among us who are suffering.

There's going to be no denying the mixture of principle and personal, fears and facts. The intent to provide compassion, dignity and autonomy by giving assisted dying is simple and amiable. But the outcry, the warnings, the objections found in the pages of submissions...

Does assisted dying really bring dignity to the dying process? Is it the only way to relieve suffering? Is it really as simple as every individual 'has a right to choose when to die'? Will this Act be sound enough to ensure security for all New Zealanders in their most vulnerable moments? Is it truly right and tight in every way?

We have a lot to consider when we put our pen to paper in the forthcoming elections? I don't want to be overly dramatic, but, for some, the way we vote could be the difference between life and death.

CHAPTER 4:

RENÉE JOUBERT

To be honest, I was expecting a hard-headed, fanatic-type person as I waded into the dogged anti-euthanasia group Euthanasia-Free NZ. But I am constantly surprised at the personal journey people have been through to get to where they stand. And at their well-thought-out and well-researched concerns and opposition.

One such person is Renée Joubert, executive officer of the organisation, who faced some of her big life questions on death when her best friend committed suicide at age 22. Renée was 20 at the time and the experience sent her into an existential crisis for several years where she questioned life and death. "During that time, I started reading on euthanasia and saw it could be one of the next big ethical dilemmas society would face," she says.

In 2013 she visited her sister in Europe. They planned to meet in Brussels, Belgium. "I thought, 'What's in Brussels? Oh, euthanasia is legal there; maybe I could talk to someone there about it'."

Renée met a doctor, a chaplain and a representative from a bioethics organisation in Belgium. The encounter thrust her into a personal journey of conviction. She connected with Euthanasia-Free NZ and soon after returning signed up to do voluntary work for them.

Renée is quick to reply to questions and it's very apparent she's fiercely opposed to this law. Her South African accent only adds to her vehemency.

"Part of what I heard in Belgium is how the culture changed as a result of their euthanasia law. That freaked me out. The Belgian oncologist I spoke to said when the law was first introduced people tended to request euthanasia in the last days of life. But 10 years later, the growing trend was to request it at their first appointment with the doctor." She says while it was intended as a last resort, in practice it just isn't.

It's probably a good time to mention we aren't the first nation to consider assisted dying laws. Since 2015 there have been 13 countries or states legalising similar laws including Canada, nine states in America, nine states in America and two in Australia, namely Victoria and Western Australia. They joined a handful of others in Europe that had adopted them like the Netherlands, Belgium, and Luxembourg. However, more than 30 jurisdictions have rejected them during this time, including the UK, 26 states in America and New South Wales in Australia.

"In the beginning I thought things were clear-cut around eligibility and process—but the longer I looked, the more I realised the lines are blurry," Renée says.

She refers to both international law and our own Act. "For example, if the goal is to alleviate suffering—does a person with a prognosis of six months to live suffer any more than a person with 10 years to live? It's inconsistent to allow euthanasia for one person suffering and not others who are suffering too. The eligibility is arbitrary."

"In the beginning I thought things were clear-cut around eligibility and process—but the longer I looked, the more I realised the lines are blurry."

Renée fears that terminal illness doesn't have the neat boundary around it that some people think it has. In Oregon, USA, "six months to live" is interpreted as, "six months to live if the person doesn't receive medical treatment". "A person could be an insulin-dependent diabetic with years or decades to live. But they could decide to stop insulin and instantly become terminal with only weeks to live."

I catch myself fumbling around with the terms 'euthanasia' and 'assisted dying' or 'assisted suicide'. Renée seems the perfect person to ask what's the difference.

The poll revealed the more strongly the person supported assisted dying, the more likely they were confused about what it means.

She says: "There are a lot of euphemisms in this field. In the end the accurate wording comes down to the actual practice. Euthanasia is when another person takes the final action; the most common method is a lethal injection. Assisted suicide is when the person accesses and administers the legal dose themselves. The most common way is either swallowed or through IV triggered by the person. Under the End of Life Choice Act the patient can choose the method they prefer."

So what is assisted dying?

"It's a euphemism. It just sounds better. Euphemisms soften it. Under current law it could be called 'culpable homicide'."

I've cautiously decided I will use 'assisted dying' as it includes both euthanasia and assisted suicide. And it's what us Kiwis are used to. But the inaccuracy of it does bother me. Confusion seems rife in this ocean of information.

In 2017 Euthanasia-Free NZ commissioned a poll asking people what they think assisted dying means. "The majority thought it means either to refuse to be resuscitated, stop treatment or turn off life support. None of those answers are correct. These choices are already legal," Renée says. "Funnily enough the poll revealed the more strongly the person supported assisted dying, the more likely they were confused about what it means. I've had this experience so many times—I'd speak to an ardent supporter of assisted dying and find out five minutes into the conversation they just don't want to be resuscitated if their heart stops."

I ask where else she sees confusion in discussions. "People like to say, 'It's my life, it's my choice'... It's sold to us as a personal choice. But it involves other people—either by making a lethal dose accessible, or by administering it. The law is about putting in place a state-administered, tax payer-funded medical treatment. It is putting a system in place to intentionally end someone's life. It involves other people."

At least one person has taken four days to die, and eight people have woken post-ingestion [after self-administering a lethal dose].

I want to know her thoughts on restoring dignity to the dying, another reason people advocate for it.

"Dignity means different things to different people. I think the way a person is cared for can restore dignity to them. I don't think a person needs to try to control their death in order to have dignity. We can't really control our own deaths anyway."

Renée says while those who support assisted dying often refer to 'bad deaths', there are a number of bad deaths that have actually been caused by the 'treatment'. "Even in euthanasia and assisted suicide there can be complications. If you think about it, it's a cocktail of drugs that is given. People's bodies react differently."

Renée is referring to reports from Oregon that show a number of complications which have happened to people who have self-administered their lethal dose. At least one person has taken four days to die, and eight people have woken post-ingestion.

"There are cases where people have had seizures, or regained consciousness, or they've passed out before they swallowed enough, or they vomited it up. It is rare, but it happens. There's no dignity in that kind of death. And I don't see how there is dignity when you are killing someone with a drug overdose.

"I want to know what people think dignity really is. Is nature not dignified? Some people say, 'I don't want someone to feed me or wipe my bum, but babies need that… Are they undignified? Some people said to me, 'It's undignified to lie for hours unconscious waiting to die'. But that's what they would go through as part of the process in euthanasia—doctors make them unconscious then administer another drug which basically gives them a heart attack."

This sort of information isn't talked about, Renée says. And she finds it disparaging that most people she speaks with don't really care or understand what's happening with euthanasia and assisted suicide overseas.

"Some people say assisted dying laws are working well overseas, but I don't think so. The review committees rely on the reports they receive from doctors and it's up to each doctor to self-report that they followed all the requirements. Of course a doctor wouldn't admit it if they've flouted a safeguard. We know from anonymous surveys that many assisted deaths are not reported, and that in these cases other requirements are often missed out too. In most jurisdictions, no independent witnesses are required when the lethal dose is administered. If the person was forced to die at that time, who would know?"

Renée's main concerns about the EOLC Act are around its lack of safeguards, such as the lack of independent witnesses needed during the final administration and when the forms are signed. And there's no mandatory cooling-off period before the lethal dose is prescribed. "The whole process, from first request to actual death, could happen in three days. This doesn't protect people from emotional decision-making."

Surely the people asking for this know what they want, and know what death is? Yet most other laws operating overseas have cooling-off periods included.

"In Oregon, there has to be an oral request, a written request and a second oral request after a waiting period of 15 days before a prescription can be written. An exception is made if the person is expected to die of their illness within that time. In Hawaii, it is 20 days.

"Under this Act someone could request euthanasia at their first appointment when they are diagnosed with a terminal illness, be seen immediately by a second doctor and the whole decision and plan be set in place. The only wait time is at least 48 hours to notify the registrar so the forms can be checked."

"The real reason why terminally-ill people want to die could be because of mental illness, not the illness that's actually killing them. And if that is the reason, they need help to live, not to die."

Renée is astonished the EOLC Act doesn't weed out those suffering from mental illness applying for assisted dying; it only considers mental 'competency' as important. "The Act clearly states that a person would not be eligible based on mental illness alone, however a terminally-ill person who is also suffering from depression or mental illness will not be excluded on that ground." That's a tragic reality considering New Zealand's huge mental health crisis, Renée says.

Also, there is no requirement for the person to be mentally competent at the time the lethal dose is administered, like the Canadian law requires. "The real reason why terminally-ill people want to die could be because of mental illness, not the illness that's actually killing them. And if that is the reason, they need help to live, not to die."

Renée says she was suicidal for over a year after her best friend died. "My dad was a GP and we were living in the same house yet he didn't know. It can be very easy to hide."

How influential is depression in those using assisted dying?

Renée says she gets emails and phone calls from people with incurable or terminal conditions who say they are depressed and want to die. They tell her they just can't get themselves to the point of killing themselves, so they want a doctor to do it. "Because we are called 'Euthanasia-Free NZ' some people think we offer a free euthanasia service..." We chuckle, but it's a bit sadistic.

"The voice of the terminally ill says 'I want to live every breath'. The voice of the well says 'my body, my choice'."

When I think about a person with a terminal illness considering assisted dying I can't help but wonder if the 'black dog' is always not far away.

"There's something called 'understandable depression' and it's common for elderly, disabled and terminally-ill people to go through this—of course they would go through it... it's part of being human. They experience a grief process, with feelings like shock, denial, anger, sadness, hopelessness, meaninglessness and, often, depression. It's just an example of things not being clear-cut. People can be in denial about their own mental space."

We wrap up our time together and Renée finishes with a saying: "The voice of the terminally ill says 'I want to live every breath'. The voice of the well says 'my body, my choice'. The fear of dying is natural. But when people deal with the fear and get the care and support they need, the most natural thing is to want to live."

CHAPTER 5:

MARY PANKO

Mary Panko is ever-ready to talk about assisted dying. Her likeable and relatable manner makes it easy to talk about her experiences and motivation behind supporting the End of Life Choice Act.

She is the president of the End-of-Life Choice Society, and while Mary is small in stature and slight in frame, you shouldn't underestimate her determination and feistiness on the issues. The retired Unitec education and technology lecturer spends many of her weekends at markets across Auckland snagging passers-by to talk about assisted dying.

Mary says she was reeled in to the issue in a similar way as me—through a friend. Her friend was terminally ill and wanted access to assisted dying. "My friend decided she wanted to have the ability to stop it all when things got too dreadful. She was desperately distraught that she had no control over her life. It laid a heavy burden on her shoulders. It wasn't legal here so she ordered the drugs online from Mexico. The drugs got stopped at customs. She died six weeks later."

Mary felt she should pay homage to her friend by finding out a bit more about assisted dying so she attended a society meeting. "I got embedded in it. The more I found out about it, the more reasonable it seemed to be for those people who wanted it."

Two more friends died who wanted access to assisted dying. "This isn't for people who are depressed, but for people who are at the end of their lives in uncontrollable pain."

Mary says research shows there are around six per cent of people who experience untreatable suffering in their last few days before death. "And in the last 24 hours before death it is much higher."

> **"This isn't for people who are depressed, but for people who are at the end of their lives in uncontrollable pain."**

What kind of suffering?

"Well, suffering in any or all forms—physically, emotionally, psychologically, spiritually. Take bowel cancer for example, it's quite a common illness. Near the end you vomit or hiccup faeces because your intestines become blocked. That is suffering. If you have emphysema your lungs fill up with fluid and you choke near death—it's as if you're drowning."

While most people won't suffer in this way, some will, she says.

"We aren't arguing that this should be introduced so people can line up for it, but it's so that the small per cent who get approved and want it can use it. The more I read and the more people I spoke to about cases where people were dying badly, the more important it became."

Originally there were two end-of-life societies in New Zealand that were set up to persuade politicians euthanasia and assisted suicide are needed. The groups joined together and redirected efforts to become an advocacy group for people who wanted access to it. The number of members is confidential.

I ask Mary if the group is happy with the End of Life Choice Act. "Yes. We are in favour of it."

I ask whether the society was disappointed at the amendments made and criteria removed from its original form. "I will say again we are in favour of the Act. We aren't going to argue any of the principles."

And Mary believes for many years the vote of the public has been supportive also. Many people she speaks to are positive and say they're all for it. "When I have been approaching people at markets to publicise medically-assisted dying there is the occasional person who rolls their eyes and walks away but a lot sign up and want to be supporters."

I ask Mary if she thinks most of the people she speaks to know much about assisted dying and the Act. "It varies hugely from what people know. When you've been involved in this issue as long as I have you think everybody knows as much as you do… but people say to me 'what referendum?'. There's a huge mixture. I was at the Takapuna market a few weeks ago and a guy stopped and asked me what I was doing, he said he is a doctor and a Muslim. He said, 'We don't need this Act... it's something doctors do anyway, they don't ask people, they just do it'. I thought—that's the whole point. People need to be asked and their choice needs to be considered."

"The more I read and the more people I spoke to about cases where people were dying badly, the more important it became."

Mary says the society is in support of palliative care in New Zealand as a whole. "Palliative care is a wonderful system and we want to see more funds invested in it. We aren't opposed to it, but the people who started it originally were often quite religious. They felt one should be calm and able to get to a spiritual conclusion near the end-of-life, and it's very Christian to give this sort of care to people. So in New Zealand they as a group oppose any form of assisted dying, which is unfortunate—although individual palliative care nurses may support it."

Mary is referring to Hospice and the Care Alliance, a group of organisations set up to focus on end-of-life care. "If you're receiving palliative care and you get to the point where you are not able to have your agony controlled you should be able to move to the other option [assisted dying]. If your abdomen is full of cancerous tissue and cells leak out—they don't have a treatment for that; it's nonsense to pretend they do. Physically palliative care can't help every case."

If assisted dying is the obvious choice to bring relief, I ask Mary why so many stand against it. "To be honest, if a person is opposed I don't bother to argue. I have previously. I've been to many meetings organised by those in opposition, and had politicians like Maggie Barry screaming at me. A large number of the audience at those meetings are very Christian. They come in bus loads to the meetings. They are told, and truly believe, it is wrong ethically and morally."

"We do not call assisted dying 'murder'. Nor would we call it 'murder' when a compassionate act helping a person to die is done at their request. The medical practitioner relieves irremediable suffering in a person nearing death— that is not murder."

So religious groups are the strongest opposition. But Mary says not all Christians are in agreement about that. One of her friends who advocated for assisted dying was a Methodist minister. He died just before Christmas in 2019. "The last few weeks of his life were filled with vomiting. It was awful. His personal point of view was he believed God was compassionate."

Mary refers me to a text another Christian advocate and former president of the society Dr Jack Havill has written which explains Christians know one of the ten commandments states that: Thou shalt not kill. "But the interpretation of this phrase according to linguistic experts is actually 'thou shalt not murder'."

A number of Bible translations now include this wording, recognising its distinction from killing. "Murder implies malevolence, is totally unwanted, and illegal," says Jack in a letter to the editor in the *NZ Herald*.

But killing can occur in legitimate circumstances, Mary says. "We do not call assisted dying 'murder'. Nor would we call it 'murder' when a compassionate act helping a person to die is done at their request. The medical practitioner relieves irremediable suffering in a person nearing death—that is not murder."

She says the current law of the land is you get treatment if you're lucky. "The aim is to keep people alive, or do no harm. If you're busy keeping people alive who don't want to be, it's harming them. There's a difference between someone begging to die less painfully and the amount of medication and treatment being incredibly invasive. We are just asking to have that stopped, and pain alleviated, and to die consciously."

Mary says palliative care doctors use terminal sedation now anyway. That's something doctors never acknowledge, she says. "When doctors carry out terminal sedation they withdraw treatment before a person is unconscious. If they choose to wake them up they are 10 times worse than before sedation because all of their treatment and pain relief has been stopped."

Mary wouldn't ever want her daughter or family to ever see her in that condition at the end of her life. "I don't want them to remember me like that. It's horrendous. If you feel like that's horrendous you should have the choice. Just like you can have the choice to live to the end without it. That's your choice. It's about giving people the right of decision."

And you believe doctors who don't want to participate also have the right to object too? "Yes. If a doctor disagrees with it I wouldn't wish them to be involved. We are only involving doctors who are willing to take part. But research done by Australian State of Victoria's Dr Nick Carr shows that there is an increase in the number of doctors willing to."

Around 327 underwent training within the first six months the practice was legal in Victoria. "Initially doctors say they don't want to, but by offering training and observation they find a larger number sign up."

However, it is noteworthy that Victoria's law only allows for assisted suicide—not euthanasia. Doctors prescribe the drug but only assist in the actual act if the person can't physically do it themselves.

"My own doctor is a Catholic and said she wouldn't do it. I didn't expect she would. If you're talking about six per cent of people suffering, and 30,000 die each year, only a tiny portion of that number are going to want it."

So if Mary has to ask for a doctor who would be willing, but the doctor doesn't know her at all, how would they be able to detect if any pressure or coercion is happening that may be influencing the decision? "Well, honestly, the doctors may not know this, but under the Act they have to enquire with the family or they could check with nursing staff. Nurses will be vital in detecting coercion: they are the ones who hear the families talking; they sit with the patients and treat them. That is the way I believe you could find out whether coercion is happening for sure."

And if the nurse refuses to participate? "Usually there is a group of nurses that see a person, but if they all refused they would speak to someone who knows the patient. Doctors can subtly ask family members, and listen. That's what doctors are trained to do."

Mary says it's a fact that if there's any evidence of people being coerced the whole thing is called off. "There are no examples abroad of coercion being practised."

Currently coercion into receiving treatment is far more prevalent, says Mary. "Families that are so-called 'loving' coerce people to live when they don't want to. That doesn't get talked about. When terminal patients want to stop and ask to stop, but a few days later come back and accept treatment, it's because their kids told them to. What is more tragic is the cases in Canada where people have had to leave their hospice facility and go outside to be assessed by doctors because the facility refused to provide it. One person on Vancouver Island who was begging for assisted dying was taken to the funeral home and received in the corridor of the funeral home. It was because they were having problems with the residential places resisting it."

Mary says it's an argument that will happen in New Zealand and will need to get sorted out. To what level can an institution refuse its involvement? "To me, that's not the same as an individual vote of conscientious objection."

"I've thought a lot about the 'slippery slope', and if it would happen... I am only fighting for the current Act, not some future [application] we cannot predict."

If assisted dying were legalised would more people want access to it than those who would be allowed? Would the law need to change?

"I've thought a lot about the 'slippery slope', and if it would happen... I am only fighting for the current Act, not some future [application] we cannot predict. People put a lot of weight in that argument. But really they are all fundamentally opposed to step one. That is their argument for stopping at the beginning. The Act we have—the one we are voting for now—is about terminal illness."

The assisted dying concept has actually been around for a while. Traces of the concept date back to pre-World War I. But one of the living founding fathers is an Australian called Philip Nitschke. He now resides in the Netherlands and runs Exit International.

Philip was the first doctor in the world to administer a legal, lethal voluntary injection. He still hosts workshops on the subject, and held several in New Zealand in 2018. But interestingly, Philip isn't a fan of our Act, tagging the legislation as "beg and grovel"... He advocates for "open access" to euthanasia.

"Don't get the idea you are in control [of life], because you are not," Philip said during one of his seminars held in New Zealand in 2018. "We believe in the human rights model, which is a right for you to dispose of your life. You have every right to give it away in a reliable and peaceful fashion. Every person should have this choice. Everyone here should make sure that you know how to end your own life now. Know how to do it and get what you need to do it. Get the drugs and put them safely aside in a cupboard because then you are in control. You will be the one who makes the decision."

CHAPTER 6:

CLAIRE FREEMAN

“Personal Account

One person who is well acquainted with Philip Nitschke’s and other overseas assisted suicide services is Claire Freeman. Claire is a 42-year-old quadriplegic and has considered travelling to Switzerland for assisted suicide to relieve her own suffering.

I’ve been looking forward to meeting Claire Freeman after watching a feature of her on TV1’s current affairs programme *Sunday*. She’s a bit of an intrigue, and one that doesn’t fit neatly into a stereotype.

On some level Claire and Lecretia Seales have a lot in common: young, intelligent, attractive, assertive… Claire, too, has faced extremely difficult circumstances and suffering. And while she doesn’t have a terminal illness, Claire is well acquainted with being near death and the challenges surrounding the EOLC Act. Before the grievous and irremediable illness clause was taken out of the eligibility criteria, she would have been granted access to assisted dying if she had applied. And even now Claire says she can very easily become eligible if she wanted to by refusing treatment and care.

I’ve struck it lucky that Claire is stopping over at the Cordis Hotel in central Auckland for a weekend after visiting her dad in Whangārei and heading home to Christchurch on Monday.

It's always a little awkward to meet someone you feel you know quite well purely through observation. I feel the need to honestly talk about myself to equal up the level of intimacy already bared.

Claire and her mum are sitting at a table on the 'high ground' of the hotel restaurant. "I'm not sitting in the 'pit of doom' as there is no ramp to get down there," says Claire, pointing over the balcony into the sunken circular lounge below. It's true, there is no access for her to order food or pay at the counter. "It would surprise you how often this actually happens," she says.

For those who haven't read her story or watched Claire on TV, she is wheelchair-bound. Claire has some movement in her arms and hands, and displays an air of sophistication. She is beautiful. Claire has caught the eye of model scouts and landed jobs on runways internationally, wheelchair and all. But it has not been an easy road. Claire has been open about her attempts of suicide after a horrendous car crash when she was 17 that changed her life forever.

"We all assumed it would get better. But it didn't. I couldn't imagine living my life in a wheelchair and not being able to use my arms. So I took a lot of pills and ended up in hospital in a coma."

Claire's mum was driving the car and fell asleep at the wheel. The car flipped and Claire sustained a spinal cord injury, losing control of her arms, hands and legs. She spent seven months in Auckland Hospital. "We all assumed it would get better. But it didn't. I couldn't imagine living my life in a wheelchair and not being able to use my arms. So I took a lot of pills and ended up in hospital in a coma."

That was her first attempted suicide. In the years that followed Claire struggled to sleep properly and threw herself into work to take her mind off it. She also studied. Claire tried to commit suicide again.

After the fourth attempt Claire went to a suicide outreach clinic. It's there that she started to talk about assisted suicide. "Both the psychologist and the psychiatrist suggested I explore assisted suicide in places overseas such as Switzerland. They didn't ask me about my lifestyle, my coping mechanisms... it was just: 'she has a broken neck, she can't move, why would she want to live?' What I didn't realise was that it wasn't my broken neck that was the problem: it's just that I didn't have the skills to cope."

"They didn't ask me about my lifestyle, my coping mechanisms... it was just: 'she has a broken neck, she can't move, why would she want to live?'"

Claire had surgery to stabilise metal work in her neck but it went badly. She was in the worst pain in her life and she lost more movement. That forced her to stop. And sleep. "I actually started reflecting on my life and lifestyle. I realised it wasn't my disability that was the problem but all the stuff manifesting in my head."

After battling depression and grief at the loss of the future she wanted, Claire has learned to run again—at least metaphorically speaking. She has a degree in design, is studying for a PhD, and owns her home in Pegasus Bay, Christchurch. And although the woman sitting in front of me looks young, she has lived a long life.

It's coffee all round as Claire admits she had a 'big night out' catching up with a male model acquaintance who had been diagnosed with a degenerative eye disease. He is going blind. From the many stories that follow it becomes clear that Claire likes to take care of those who 'don't fit in boxes' and she gives hope to the down-and-out. I have a lot of questions for Claire and I know she will have insight and personal experience to add.

"I was at a dinner table with politicians and pro-euthanasia people and they all said 'One of the worst things in the world would be having someone wipe your bum'. So I stopped them and said: 'Well, speaking from personal experience, I've had people wipe my arse and I can tell you something—it's really not as bad as you think.' They looked at me oddly. There's irrational fear at play in this discussion, and I get why we have that fear, but we need to break down some of these discourses."

"I was at a dinner table with politicians and pro-euthanasia people and they all said 'One of the worst things in the world would be having someone wipe your bum'. So I stopped them and said: 'Well, speaking from personal experience, I've had people wipe my arse and I can tell you something—it's really not as bad as you think.'"

Claire says she isn't an anti-euthanasia campaigner—she just doesn't think we as a society are at a stage where we can make decisions around assisted dying in an "unbiased and ethically-informed manner".

So, what are our existing biases? "I think people's perception around euthanasia is based on fear. Fear of a concept of dignity, which is based on independence. It's this individualist culture of not wanting to have people look after you."

Claire's father had a stroke last year and was given a grim prognosis. "When Dad was in a critical condition our family met with the health professionals who said if he pulls out of the coma his quality of life will be so poor that they recommended not to continue treatment."

Claire asked what kind of quality of life they meant. "They said he would probably have to use a wheelchair and they were pretty sure there was brain damage. They said he's quite old, and he's had a good life."

The family agreed for treatment to continue and Claire's dad survived much of what was predicted but, among other things, he can no longer walk. Before the incident he was a scientist and was fiercely independent.

"The sad thing is Dad doesn't want us to see him being disabled, which is ironic considering I'm disabled. My sister went and looked after him for respite care. She said the crazy thing is, 'Yes, I had to wipe his arse and I had to put nappies on him and stuff, but we had a talk about it. And actually when I was doing it, it was quite an intimate time between us.'" Her sister explained that the initial difficulty quickly changed to a closeness, a journey that demonstrated the truth about dignity.

Claire says not only are people afraid of the unknown and dying itself, but also of losing what they call "dignity"... which is actually just the quality of life they are used to.

Controversial Australian philosopher Peter Singer discusses the validity of euthanasia based on a person's quality of life, Claire says. "He makes the assumption essentially that if you are disabled or critically ill you have no quality of life. There's no point where their life will get better; that's why they should have that option of assisted dying."

"When someone is a vegetable or may not have cognitive abilities—we can look and assume we know what their life is like, but we don't. There is always value in life."

To Claire, that's an arrogant way to think. Her life story demonstrates the opposite. "It's as if the value of someone's life is measured on this scale of 'function'. That perception is active in the medical field today.

I know through research that 80 per cent of healthcare professionals wouldn't want to live with my condition."

"It's the dark times of suffering that makes life richer and more beautiful. "Suffering isn't a bad thing. It's a learning experience. You have to choose to embrace the life you have or you will never be at peace or find joy or see the purpose."

These are the same professionals who will be gate-keeping assisted dying.

"When someone is a vegetable or may not have cognitive abilities—we can look and assume we know what their life is like, but we don't. There is always value in life. It's the most profound thing. Life is magical because you can't explain it. It's a difficult concept to get your head around."

Claire says it's the dark times of suffering that makes life richer and more beautiful. "Suffering isn't a bad thing. It's a learning experience. You have to choose to embrace the life you have or you will never be at peace or find joy or see the purpose."

To be honest, I'd find it hard to receive this message from anyone else but Claire. It's really only because she has had to choose to turn pain and suffering into something beautiful herself. Claire says the reality is that if assisted dying were available in New Zealand she would be dead.

Claire fits the description that promoters say this treatment is for—someone well educated, determined, financially secure. But she says those things don't provide immunisation from vulnerability. "I'm sure there are probably an awful lot of people who might choose it that wouldn't classify themselves as vulnerable. But, to be honest, the term 'vulnerable' is interesting in itself. Many people say it's patronising. I don't think it is. It's just part of life. I'm fine calling myself vulnerable—we all are in some situations. If you can admit it, it actually puts you in a more powerful position."

I ask Claire if she means the ones who will elect to use it are vulnerable in a more non-traditional sense of the word. "Yes, I think so. They've been subjected to the different discourses we've had about death and dying. They have just found out they are dying. And there will be those who are vulnerable in the same way I am—they will still be caught in the crossfire. There is collateral damage that comes from this, even if they aren't a big chunk of the statistics."

That collateral damage should be prevented by safeguards and eligibility limitations. But Claire thinks these wont do the job. "The law changes; it expands—it does. You just have to look into the application of the law in the other nations that have this. I do believe in the eventuality of people like myself being included in this."

And when that expansion happens Claire is worried for those who will be left unprotected. If the option of assisted dying is available many who have faced tragic situations like hers will choose it. "I see just about everyone who has a spinal cord injury in the country, and for two to five years they are highly suicidal. They would choose this. And that makes me really angry. It's a hell of a shock [when you get injured]. It's terrifying, but it gets better. And you can move past that. These people will not be given the opportunity to

"It's a hell of a shock [when you get injured]. It's terrifying, but it gets better. And you can move past that. These people will not be given the opportunity to grieve, have support, and know life gets better... It's our job to protect them."

"We could be creating a very homogenised, boring world because we aren't protecting the people who make this world an interesting place."

grieve, have support, and know life gets better… It's our job to protect them.

"I just don't know how we got to this point—if we are going to stigmatise mental health in that way. I'm not saying to live with these issues is easy, because it's not. But on the other hand, it also gives you values and skills you wouldn't otherwise have."

Claire says there's serious potential that we would lose the lives of great and influential people because this law would open the door for premature death. "Da Vinci, Mozart... so many great people in history had mental health issues. If we had this law back then it's entirely possible they wouldn't be here. We could be creating a very homogenised, boring world because we aren't protecting the people who make this world an interesting place, who think outside the square, even when people look at us [in a wheelchair] and say 'not my cup of tea'. I know in myself I have something to give because of what I've been through. I hope that creates some change in the world; I want to give something. And that's exciting for me."

Claire has had to journey through the grief, loss, anger and frustration, and create a new normal—one that is worth living. So it's no surprise why she is vested in this if it threatens those who will find themselves in her shoes. But how does she weigh this with giving people the right to make their own choices? I ask her how she interprets 'it's my life, my choice'.

"I think it's a massive reflection on our culture and society. I think it's a naive and sad idea. Although on one level it makes sense and sounds fantastic, and we all want choice and to be free, but it's just not that black and white. I feel like it's really superficial. I wish people would think about it a bit more. Choice is something we all want. It's seductive, beautiful, intoxicating. But choice comes with baggage."

Claire says she would be sitting next to David Seymour championing the Act up until around three years ago. She wanted to use it for herself for nearly 20 years. "In hindsight it was just because I wasn't coping with life. What I realised is that I didn't have the support. The problem is that people with disabilities don't have the right support. We need to ensure they do before we even entertain the thought of a law like this—otherwise, there isn't really a choice at all."

Claire says the elephant in the room that people never talk about in relation to assisted dying is the economy. "The cost of keeping people like myself alive. As part of my PhD research it keeps coming up—people can't get a powered wheelchair because it costs too much… It's not discussed.

"Look, the concept of assisted suicide is a good one—having choice and dignity is a beautiful thing. But as human beings I don't feel we are ready; we don't understand it enough to put it in practice. Putting it in place now is horrendously dangerous."

Speaking of the economy, I need to pay for our drinks down in the 'pit of doom' below. As we finish up I ask Claire why she thinks us Kiwis don't talk much about death, disability and struggles… How do we get past our reservedness? "We need to

Claire says the elephant in the room that people never talk about in relation to assisted dying is the economy. "The cost of keeping people like myself alive. As part of my PhD research it keeps coming up—people can't get a powered wheelchair because it costs too much... It's not discussed."

"We are scrambling to find out why we have such a high suicide rate. We want to make it better, and we want to address why it is happening. How can we not see that the two issues have huge similarities? Assisted dying—it's a request to kill yourself. We are saying it is OK if they are terminal. It's inconsistent."

address Kiwi culture. Seeing other cultures like even Spanish culture—people are more open to talk about things. Kiwis have a very conservative way of looking at things and we don't like conflict, so we shy away from it.

"We are scrambling to find out why we have such a high suicide rate. We want to make it better, and we want to address why it is happening. How can we not see that the two issues have huge similarities? Assisted dying—it's a request to kill yourself. We are saying it is OK if they are terminal. It's inconsistent. People just don't want to think about the bad stuff. It's too dark. We need to think about how to put it in a way that's palatable so we can talk about it."

The beast of suffering. It can touch everything, and it threatens to heed nothing. It affects everybody, and pardons nobody. It's unliked and uncomfortable. We want to lessen it, contain it, or eradicate it. But it seems to be bound to life, just as love is to risk.

Claire's perspective on the obsession of extinguishing suffering is challenging. If we remove suffering completely we would lose the shadows which contrast the light; we would lose the winters and the nights. However difficult or inconvenient or exhausting or unjust... there is still good to be found in it.

I know that could perhaps sound insensitive to someone presently walking through suffering. But however difficult, it still holds true. That's what hope is, right? An expectation of good.

SECTION 3:

MEDICAL PERSPECTIVES

Medical practitioners carry a heavy weight of responsibility in the world we live in. They intervene, treat and save lives on a daily basis. They're real-life superheroes. But in return we have high expectations of them. They are the ones we turn to when our bodies give way. The ones we rely on when we don't know what's wrong. And they are the ones on the frontline of this issue.

Every doctor or medical professional I have spoken to about assisted dying has said the same thing. They don't really like talking about it. They don't like to raise their heads on controversial social issues. It's just not natural to their nature. So when thousands of them have signed petitions, drafted submissions and fronted up to the media against the issue it is a surprising phenomena in itself.

I think their speaking up is warranted. They will be the ones prescribing the lethal dose, injecting the needle in someone's arm and implementing the final push off into eternity for their patients if the EOLC Act is passed. In the words of Clint Eastwood in the film Unforgiven: "It's a helluva thing, killing a man. You take away all he's got and he's ever gonna have."

The medical world is a bit of a microcosm. It has its own set of values, processes, culture and systems. I think it's fair to say that most of us experience them, but not many of us understand them. I'm taking an exploratory mission probing into the enigma of healthcare to see where it interfaces with assisted dying.

One of the gatekeepers of all things medical is The New Zealand Medical Association (NZMA). It's the country's only pan-professional medical organisation with around 5,000 members that represents the collective interests of all doctors. Its job is to advocate on medico-political issues, providing leadership to the medical profession to promote ethics, unity, values and the health of all New Zealanders. And their stance on assisted dying is fairly hard-hitting:

"The NZMA is opposed to euthanasia and doctor-assisted suicide. We regard these practices to be unethical and harmful to individuals, especially vulnerable people, and society. Accordingly, we do not support the proposed End of Life Choice Act," their select committee submission says.

"The Act doesn't address the social issues—particularly those of coercion, competence and vulnerability."

"Furthermore, we believe the Act itself has a number of serious shortcomings and technical flaws. These reflect the impossibility of drafting euthanasia and doctor-assisted suicide legislation that is completely effective in terms of defining those eligible, ensuring a free choice, protecting the vulnerable, and ensuring competency.

"In conclusion, euthanasia in any form conflicts with the ethical principles of medical practice and would change the fundamental role of the doctor and the doctor/patient relationship."

NZMA chairperson Dr Kate Baddock added: "The Act doesn't address the social issues—particularly those of coercion, competence and vulnerability. It does not protect the vulnerable, the weak, the lonely, those in pain and suffering; it doesn't protect them from wrongful death. We don't believe any law can be crafted that could do so."

Her statement is an early indicator of the atmospheric conditions ahead.

Something you need to know… In upcoming chapters you will find the word 'safeguard' referred to a number of times. Safeguard is the name given by David Seymour to specific processes in place that were included to protect individuals from potential hazards of the law. These are such things as doctors required to do their best to ensure no coercion has influenced someone's decision, therefore providing a safeguard against potential abuse. Why are the safeguards important? Well, they are really the only things standing in the way of this law being used for evil instead of good. And when we are talking about life and death, everyone agrees the safeguards need to work.

Ready to launch.

CHAPTER 7:

DR SINÉAD DONNELLY

It's a bit of a game of cat and mouse getting Dr Sinéad Donnelly on the phone for an interview. Understandably she's incredibly busy as she works as a general medicine physician at Wellington Hospital. She is also a clinical associate professor of palliative medicine at Otago University and produces extensive research publications on general medicine-related topics. But her opinion on this issue is absolutely critical. I want to hear from the doctors who will be directly affected by this law.

I finally pin her down. "Hi, Sinéad. Have I got you at a good time?"... A quiet Irish voice speaks back to me. She is soft, but certain. Pleasantries exchanged, I asked her why she had waded in on this issue. "I am the doctor potentially injecting this drug. I have to be for, or against. I can't abstain from this," she points out.

I wonder if Sinéad would ever be one who would put herself out there to speak to the media, represent 1,500 other doctors, or conduct interviews like this one, if it weren't being thrust upon her.

Sinéad was one of the people behind the Doctors Say No campaign, an open letter to politicians and policymakers stating doctors want no part in euthanasia and assisted suicide, and, among other things, that the practice was unethical even if it were made legal. I'd been waiting to ask a doctor this question… Can you tell me the difference between a diagnosis and prognosis, and how accurate are prognoses anyway?

"I am the doctor potentially injecting this drug. I have to be for, or against. I can't abstain from this."

"Diagnosis is saying what illness you have. Like you go for a test and find you have the coronavirus. That's what's wrong with you. The prognosis is how you are going to do. Like 'you may get better but it will take a few days'. And we make those assessments based on your age, how healthy you are, any previous illnesses, things like that… but it still has an element of guesswork involved."

From what I had read so far, it seemed a six-month terminal prognosis was too shifty to peg eligibility for requested death on it. What does Sinéad think?

"We consider prognostication as an art not a science. It's a guess. The literature around this topic says that our chances of being right within hours, or a day or two... we could possibly figure that out. But not months. It becomes far less accurate. It's impossible to say someone definitely has six months to live."

And because of this Sinéad says it is definitely not a safeguard like the EOLC Act suggests. "If you could plug facts and information into a computer about a person and it comes up with a complete and accurate analysis and a date they will die, well then you could make that a law. But every person is different."

International reports support this reality. According to *The American Journal of Medicine*, 11 published studies indicate misdiagnosis occurs anywhere from 10 to 15 per cent of the time. The US State of Washington Death With Dignity Act Report annually records information about everyone who has requested assisted suicide in the state. Washington State offers assisted suicide only as an option and patients take the drug home with them and ingest it when they want to. It's law also includes the six-month terminal prognosis criteria. The results are interesting. In the five years from 2013 to 2018 a total of 116 people who had requested assisted suicide lived longer than six months. Some lived years longer. And that number doesn't even take into consideration those who chose to end their lives early. Who knows how many would live beyond the six months given to them by doctors?

I don't know if it brings relief or concern that prognosis is that inaccurate—it will certainly make me think twice about ending my life on a doctor's report if I ever get a bad one. It also makes me seriously question whether we should be using this as a measurement.

According to *The American Journal of Medicine*, 11 published studies indicate misdiagnosis occurs anywhere from 10 to 15 per cent of the time.

"There's a number of concerns I have about the EOLC Act like this," Sinéad says. "Like the fact it will directly impact the patient/doctor relationship. When euthanasia is on the table a patient will say, 'I wish it was all over and I want euthanasia'. If this law is passed no longer will we be allowed to engage with the patient in a normal therapeutic way and say, 'let's explore that and work deeply'. We're required to move along once they have requested it, into the process. We are no longer professionals using our clinical judgement—we're technicians."

Sinéad says when patients explain they've had enough of life she gently and carefully explores why. "After many years of experience I know this approach works. The greatest need in my experience is for people to be truly heard and listened to, not abandoned.

"I recently had a 48-year-old lady who had been diagnosed with widespread cancer, which took two years and much distress to diagnose, say to me: 'This is all too much....'. I asked her what was too much. Going to hospital? Did she not want the chemotherapy? She replied,

'Oh, I do; I do want the treatment. I just want to be cared for with kindness. For someone to bring me a cigarette, give me a wheat pack, make me a cup of Milo.'"

"It's the destruction of the doctor/patient relationship. It will destroy the heart and soul of medicine."

That concept of care has been built into Sinéad's genes as a third-generation doctor. "The idea of intentionally ending someone's life, the very concept is heartbreaking for me. The thought that doctors I work with or teach, the medical students I am educating—that their future may include them intentionally killing someone's life. It's the destruction of the doctor/patient relationship. It will destroy the heart and soul of medicine."

Sinéad is adamant that the line has to be held. "The doctor doesn't intentionally cause harm. We have zero tolerance for that in our profession. That's what medicine pivots on. If society insists it wants the ability to end people's lives—this may sound selfish and I suppose it is—then the medical profession doesn't have to be involved.

"Don't use the cloak of medicine to provide legitimacy for this. The other name this action would be given is to kill someone. We need to take the protective cloak of medicine away from what is in fact deliberately ending the life of another person."

Strong sentiment held by Sinéad isn't necessarily shared across all doctors. But the Act has included a clause called "conscientious objection" as a safeguard to protect doctors who object for personal reasons. This would work, right?

"Well, who will actually do it [euthanasia] then? Another doctor. We actually really care about the people we look after. Even if you opt out you will still see the person in the same hospital or practice being treated by doctors who choose to do it. We have been doctors to some patients for decades… Treated both them and their children and grandchildren. This still has a big impact on us."

Objecting doctors must refer patients who request assisted dying on to the SCENZ Group. This is considered complicit involvement, with a number of other jurisdictions not requiring this in their legislation.

Sinéad says conscientious objection options are already being challenged, and it isn't a guaranteed safeguard. I'm referred to a statement released from Oxford University's Uehiro Centre for Practical Ethics.

In June 2016 the university invited a group of philosophers and bioethicists to Geneva, Switzerland, to participate in a workshop on conscientious objection in healthcare and propose guidelines for regulation. One of the contributing members was Otago University senior lecturer in bioethics Professor Angela Ballantyne.

The first two recommendations in the guidelines included: *"Healthcare practitioners' primary obligations are towards their patients, not towards their own personal conscience. When the patient's wellbeing (or best interest, or health) is at stake, healthcare practitioners' professional obligations should normally take priority over their personal moral or religious views."*

And: *"In the event of a conflict between practitioners' conscience and a patient's desire for a legal, professionally sanctioned medical service, healthcare practitioners should always ensure that patients receive timely medical care... In emergency situations, when referral is not possible, or when it poses too great a burden on patients or on the healthcare system, health practitioners should perform the treatment themselves."*

"We need to take the protective cloak of medicine away from what is in fact deliberately ending the life of another person."

In the case of providing assisted dying as a 'healthcare service', I can see how this could be interpreted as the patient's desire for euthanasia would override the practitioner's conscientious objection when referrals are not possible.

Sinéad also points to a news article which quotes former MP and former End-of-Life Choice Society president Maryan Street saying all doctors should be compelled to provide assisted dying: "Just because they don't agree with a patient's choice they can't abandon the patient. That's unethical. That's unprofessional. That is supremely challengeable in my view."

"People yearn so much to receive care unconditionally that they are acutely sensitive to any sign of being a burden."

If Sinéad thinks a doctor's right to objection isn't a good safeguard, then what about the safeguards around protecting people from coercion?

"People yearn so much to receive care unconditionally that they are acutely sensitive to any sign of being a burden. If they sense this they close down, retreat and their pain increases. There is no doubt coercion happens in everyday life. If there's any chance that the law is weakening the protection it has to the vulnerable, it is unacceptable."

But are there safeguards to detect external pressure on the patients? "Dysfunctional ones," Sinéad says. "Also, pressure is very difficult to detect and requires a long-term relationship between doctor and patient. In Oregon in 2017, the median doctor/patient relationship before an assisted suicide prescription was just 10 weeks.

"Increasing numbers of people in Washington and Oregon have named being a burden on family and friends as one of the main reasons they opted for assisted suicide."

In the State of Washington in 2018, this was 51 per cent of the people who received a lethal prescription. In fact, inadequate pain control, or fear of it, was 38 per cent. Pain control has been cited by almost everyone advocating for assisted dying. It's a contributing factor for 'bad deaths' in New Zealand, with Mary Panko saying around six per cent of people have pain or suffering that can't be controlled by medication.

I ask Sinéad if this is true. And shouldn't they have access to assisted dying.

"Those who specialise in palliative care say they feel they have all the tools they need to attend to someone's pain. They know how to, and can, administer medication that will help. Suffering is a little more subjective: we can't say we can relieve all suffering. Yet there is a lot we can do. But when pain or suffering is too great, there are times when you can give palliative sedation. It's given in a very small percentage [of cases] and basically puts the person into a coma. But you are doing it to relieve their symptoms and let nature take its course. And it's reversible—you aren't causing death. No palliative care doctor or nurse would tolerate being in front of someone with unbearable suffering and doing nothing. There is always something we can do."

In Oregon in 2017, the median doctor/patient relationship before an assisted suicide prescription was just 10 weeks.

Sinéad says the issue is more around people getting access to good palliative care as well as a lack of funding. "There are a lot of aged residential care facilities that cater for people dying but they are businesses, so may not necessarily have good palliative care input. There are areas that could be improved."

She says the widespread confusion around what people have already got access to when it comes to end-of-life care and dying doesn't help the situation. And according to polls by Curia Market Research done in New Zealand in 2017, she is right. There seems to be some major confusion over what is already provided for or is 'legal' when it comes to end-of-life care and dying. For one, can doctors legally inject lethal amounts of morphine already?

"Well there is a misconception that morphine kills people. It doesn't. It's not an effective agent to kill. Often people who are dying are given an extra dose of morphine, but it is an appropriate dose to relieve any pain they may have… and they happen to die after."

Stopping treatment, refusing treatment, turning off life support, refusing life support and having a 'do not resuscitate' order are already legal, medically ethical, and are not euthanasia. How are they any different from euthanasia?

"It's all about the intent," Sinéad says. "The withdrawal of treatment is totally different from the doctor intentionally ending the life of a patient."

Stopping treatment, refusing treatment, turning off life support, refusing life support and having a 'do not resuscitate' order are already legal, medically ethical, and are not euthanasia.

So if we have all the resources to relieve suffering, why do so many people, including MPs, share their traumatic stories of seeing relatives die?

"There will be cases where some people don't get the care they deserve. But often the pain and grief of the people watching a person die is much greater than the one experiencing it. For the people watching the death of a loved one, they are faced with their own unexplored existential issues around dying and death. All your own fear around the mystery and pain of dying is activated because you are there; it's exploding inside of you if you haven't attended to it. You bring all your ways of coping with life to that moment. And you aren't necessarily aware.

"Then there is the grief of a loved one dying. The observer's response is very complex. In palliative care, we are attending in equal proportion to the patient and their family who is there. At times the observer is even more important. If you don't attend to someone's experience of death in a wholesome way, they will come out in a non-wholesome way of life."

"Often the pain and grief of the people watching a person die is much greater than the one experiencing it. For the people watching the death of a loved one, they are faced with their own unexplored existential issues around dying and death."

Sinéad says she thinks there are deeper reasons driving the assisted dying push. "The topic of death reaches to the ultimate core of our being. What I think is happening psychologically in this day and age is we want to fix the existential dread of the unknown and dying. I truly believe the ultimate inner core of this revolves around dread. We do different things to cope with this… One of the things is euthanasia. We don't talk about that in the public arena.

"Having control takes the edge off fear. But this has all been projected onto the issue of euthanasia and assisted dying."

Sinéad's final plea for Kiwis to consider: "If you move from a world where a doctor doesn't kill a patient, to now it does—it's a completely different world. All I think doctors [who are opposed to the Act] would ask is that people have their eyes open and listen to these ideas and consequences, and then vote. All we are asking is for a 50/50 space to explain all of this."

Before our time has concluded I want to fire a few questions to Sinéad in response to comments made by End-of-Life Choice Society

"Having control takes the edge off fear. But this has all been projected onto the issue of euthanasia and assisted dying."

president Mary Panko. Firstly, is terminal sedation a thing?

"No. Terminal is not even a medical term. What we do is palliative sedation, and it is purely the way of providing symptom control."

Do doctors withdraw treatment before putting a patient in palliative sedation—so that if and when they wake they will be worse off because the treatment and pain relief has stopped?

"That is totally incorrect. It is a case of listening to the experts, not to social media. Even the fact someone would suggest that is like a knife into me emotionally. We are there to alleviate suffering. It's never our intention to kill."

Secondly, emphysema… do people die unable to breathe and drowning in their own mucus?

"No. Technically it doesn't have anything to do with fluid. Mary is clearly not a doctor. If we were looking after a patient who had difficulty breathing, we would give them a low-dose medication that would help."

I took a night off from writing to catch up with a good friend. She happens to be a nurse. So of course our conversation went from, "How is married life?" to "How is the book going?"… As we talk through the discoveries and interviews so far, we seem to dance around the issues until finally landing on the motivation behind such laws. She can't help wonder why we run from suffering at all costs.

My friend worked on the African Mercy Ship as a volunteer nurse for several years. She recalls meeting and speaking to a mother who had lost four of her eight children to sickness, a story that is common in the nations the ship visits. Yet the woman didn't blink once in retelling her story of loss. "I felt pity for her but she was profoundly content and didn't want pity. She had found happiness in what her normal is," my friend said.

I've heard many similar stories, of people in nations of tremendous poverty and suffering having peace, contentment and joy far greater than those who are perceived as wealthy.

With modern healthcare and support in place we have tremendously reduced suffering yet in turn it seems we have sheltered ourselves from its reality. It has become a distant acquaintance rather than a close friend. Is it possible the result is that we don't know how to cope with it, how to recover from it, how to bear up under it, and we don't want to face it? In our best efforts to eliminate suffering have we in fact been weakened to it?

As a parent of young children, I know we are often told to allow your child to be exposed to germs as it actually helps build a child's immunity. Obviously this has to be done in balance. You wouldn't thrust your child into a filthy, germ-infested bathroom and not wash their hands—but some exposure is necessary. But how far should we go as humanity in exposing ourselves to struggle and adversity so as to keep us strong?

CHAPTER 8:

PROFESSOR RODERICK MACLEOD MNZM

"Palliative care is a wonderful thing, but like medicine, it is not perfect. So the question becomes: what do we do if we know that palliative care cannot deal with all suffering? Do we just accept that some people will suffer awful deaths, turn away from them and decide that those people are just unlucky? Or do we listen to them, show compassion and allow those people to have a choice about how they die? – **Matthew Vickers, husband of the late Lecretia Seales**

When I first called Professor Roderick (Rod) MacLeod his soothing tone and British accent sounded like a mix of Sir David Attenborough, Michael Caine and my dad. He is quite obviously intelligent, caring and humble.

Rod has a list of qualifications longer than the line of people in the supermarket checkout queue during the COVID-19 outbreak. He's an honoured Member of the New Zealand Order of Merit and has worked around the world researching, teaching and advising medical professionals on end-of-life care. He's currently an honoured professor at the University of Sydney Northern Clinical School and an honorary academic in palliative care at the University of Auckland, as well as a Hospice Advisor. I think I could fill a page with his CV.

Yet here he was, prepared to sit and explain the basics of what he does over the phone with me on a Friday morning. His answer to Matthew Vickers' question—invest more in palliative care.

Rod says palliative care is effective, but its main restrictions are around people having limited access and not enough funding. "Palliative care is not perfect—we have to own that. But the investment has been so limited. There are only a small number of palliative care specialists in this country and in all our big hospitals in New Zealand today, a third of people in them will be dead within a year. Why aren't there small armies of palliative care doctors, nurses and counsellors helping people to adjust to huge change?"

Rod says introducing assisted dying without improving end-of-life care is the wrong way around.

In New Zealand 50 per cent of investment in palliative care comes from the government, but the rest is from the community. "It sounds good, but imagine if someone said to you they would pay for half of your intensive care in a hospital but you have to fundraise the rest. There would be an outcry."

"It's about life and living and making the most of life, not filling people up with drugs and floating them off."

So, what is palliative care exactly? I know it involves caring for someone dying, and hospice specialises in it… but to be exact, the Ministry of Health states it involves supporting and helping a person to live as comfortably and fully as possible. It's for someone with a life-limiting illness that cannot be cured and may at some time result in the person dying. It's provided in the community, hospices and hospitals and can be provided by all healthcare professionals supported by specialist services.

"It's about life and living and making the most of life, not filling people up with drugs and floating them off," Rod says.

He explains a palliative care specialist has as much training as any other medical specialist. "You do five or six years as a med student, another two or three post-registration, then if you decide you want to be a specialist in palliative medicine, you do another three years."

"Medical students spend 12 weeks learning about the beginning of life and must observe babies being delivered, but they only receive one lecture and a day in hospice for the end-of-life training."

There's a widespread lack of palliative specialists, but what is far worse is the lack of basic training all doctors receive in palliative care. That's despite the fact a newly-minted doctor in New Zealand will care for 40 people and their families dying in their first year alone. "Medical students spend 12 weeks learning about the beginning of life and must observe babies being delivered, but they only receive one lecture and a day in hospice for the end-of-life training. It's not surprising people are frightened about death. Even doctors are."

But he says giving someone control over the timing of death is not the answer. The solution to people in fear—education. "I think fear of death is real. Most people only experience what it's like from TV or movies and there it is rarely portrayed as being gentle and kind."

Palliative care provides a preparation for people so they understand what is going to happen. "At the end-of-life we know what's going to happen and what the process is. There's specific things that happen in every person, and as a specialist we can actually see them happening. For example, near the end you get more tired. It's a way of the body shutting down and getting ready. Your breathing might change, you might spend more time sleeping but wake feeling refreshed.

"Another change we see is you start worrying less about the world, less about what's going on in New Zealand… your world shrinks. Your sense of preservation means you focus only on those closest to you. Then you end up focusing on yourself. I think that can be distressing for families, as they feel cut out. It's most often the families that get most worried at this stage." The last sense to shut down is hearing.

I wish I had Rod around when my granddad was dying. I was in hospital with Granddad after he had a stroke a couple of years ago. He was in a coma for the last few days of his life. I had very little knowledge of what was happening or why. Thankfully there weren't signs of any major distress from him, but probably the most difficult part was understanding what calls doctors and family were making around his care and medical intervention. In the end he died peacefully one night in his sleep at his rest home. Understanding the signs of dying would have helped me know what was going on and what to expect.

"People often say they are fearful of being on their own when they die of pain, or some sort of distress. All those things can be remedied," says Rod. "You won't abandon them as a carer, you can manage pain… It's not going to be so hard that you say 'let's end it now'."

Rod's solution to people in suffering and indignity—care. The concept of suffering is a difficult one and can mean a vast variety of things, he says. It's entirely subjective and at times surprising what people suffer from.

"One woman I treated had a very serious joint disease so every time her limbs moved you could hear the joints crushing. She had treatment but developed bone cancer. I asked her if she was suffering. She said, 'Yes'. So I asked if she could tell me about it. She said her son went out sailing three years ago and never came back. Her physical suffering was nothing compared to the loss of her son." So to say something like assisted dying will relieve suffering is an impossible and immeasurable goal, Rod says.

"It's also difficult to distinguish between a suffering that is ongoing and one that comes and goes. What might seem unbearable at one point no longer does at another point. It's often the fear of suffering, not the suffering itself, which is the trigger that promotes people to seek assisted dying," Rod says. "If we enquire, explore and talk about it you would find some of that six per cent might find relief. Nobody can tell you they can take suffering away. But that doesn't mean to say the remedy is to kill them. All the people I've met near the end of their life have taught me something. They've taught me that people on the whole want to live life and value it."

What does Rod think about assisted dying and the EOLC Act?

"I was teaching a group of postgraduates yesterday who were all studying palliative care. I asked them, 'How many have read the Bill?' And only one in the class of 20 put their hand up. I thought, 'Well, here are people invested in palliative care who know about it, and work in it, and yet they haven't read the bill that will directly affect them.'

"I don't know how to get people to understand that this is about a deeply flawed Act and that it is extremely dangerous."

"I don't know how to get people to understand that this is about a deeply flawed Act and that it is extremely dangerous."

He says we always hear about countries that have introduced it, but not about the many more that debated and ruled it out. Essentially it is being pushed as a European-based decision, he says. "I don't see it in Africa, South-East Asia, South American [other than Colombia], or within any Latino communities. It's something the white middle class are pushing."

Rod has a very interesting point. It seems a little elitist.

"I'm not sure why it's a European thing—maybe something to do with the disintegration of the family," Rod says. "Many of these other nations have reverence and responsibility to those who are older and more frail."

> **"There's a lot of science involved in prognostication, but really it is still an art. We know from years of practice that doctors are not good at it. They make mistakes."**

The choice of assisted dying will have an impact on everyone in society. Rod says such big decisions shouldn't be made with so little knowledge.

And a person choosing life or death shouldn't hinge their decision on an inaccurate measurement of prognosis. "There's a lot of science involved in prognostication, but really it is still an art. We know from years of practice that doctors are not good at it. They make mistakes.

"One of my first patients I cared for as a palliative care doctor was a guy who was having enormous doses of morphine regularly. He was diagnosed with a nasty malignant tumour in his bones. I thought he looked well for someone so sick. We talked and agreed to reduce the amount of painkillers. We wittled it down over time until he wasn't taking any. He said, 'They told me I was dying, that's why I was taking medication.' So we decided to get another scan to see how far the illness had progressed. To our surprise and astonishment he had no disease at all. Here was a man referred to hospice because he was dying with widespread metastatic disease, but there had been a mistake. He was absolutely stunned and lived on for years.

"I've seen a few people in my career who have been diagnosed with malignancy who haven't had it—So much so that I thought I should get a T-shirt printed that says, 'I survived hospice'. Most doctors have stories like that; it's a tiny percentage, but it happens."

Rod says his other worry is the doctor/patient relationship. "You've taken an oath you aren't going to harm, you will help them, you will try your best to help them feel better. I can't put my hand on my heart and make everyone better. But I have looked after 15,000 people and for every single one, I've tried my absolute best and most have felt better. Killing is the complete opposite of what I went into medicine for."

There have been countless times Rod has heard patients say they have had enough. "If you take a poll of people who first arrive at palliative care thinking about euthanasia it would actually be moderately high. After a couple of weeks that number will drop significantly. I can only remember one man who persisted in wanting to end his life. Each day when I asked him if I could do it (hypothetically), would it be today that he wanted it? He would always say, 'No, no, not today, but tomorrow'. He died a very peaceful death."

While Rod won't have to perform euthanasia himself he says it directly impacts on people he cares for. "It is about society and how we value people who aren't well. We are saying to some people—your life isn't worth living. I've never met anyone in my career and thought, 'You are better off dead'. Yes, there's been desperately sick people and those who are hugely sad and anxious. But that's not an excuse for ending their life—rather an opportunity to find out how as a group of professionals and society [we] can help them."

"Yes, there's been desperately sick people and those who are hugely sad and anxious. But that's not an excuse for ending their life—rather an opportunity to find out how as a group of professionals and society [we] can help them."

If assisted dying is going to be considered a medical treatment, Rod says it needs to have the same level of data available for analysis as any other field of medicine.

"The review committee is the only one that will get to see any of the statistics; we won't know any more details than the public or even the medical specialists—just the raw number who decided on it. In every area of medicine we have very accurate statistics. It's just not good enough. There's gaping holes."

Before we finish I run past Rod one of the horrible cases of dying which Mary Panko mentioned in her interview—bowel cancer leading to a person hiccupping faeces. Does it happen?

"It's a rare thing but a person can get an intestinal obstruction. They no longer get bowel motion so whatever they eat has to come out another way."

For someone in this situation one of the aims of palliative treatment would be to reduce the outpouring of fluid into the gut, Rod says. "Normally this fluid would just get absorbed but when it can't we can use drugs to reduce the amount being produced. You can cut down the amount significantly." Another option would be a venting gastrostomy but it isn't very pleasant.

> **"We are not magicians. Dying is not easy. It can be hard work because most people don't want to do it."**

He recalls a recent case involving a woman in her 40s suffering from a bowel obstruction who he had cared for. "She was determined to stay alive until her husband returned from duty in the military. Every evening she had a gin and tonic. Once a day she vomited. Her quality of life was as such that she could spend her days doing what she wanted. We were fortunate to find drugs that made her comfortable."

Rod says specialists do their best and never give up trying to reduce a problem for their patients. "But we are not magicians. Dying is not easy. It can be hard work because most people don't want to do it."

Coming away from an interview with Rod makes me realise what an honour it is to have people like him dedicating their lives to study and giving thousands of hours to care for people near death. The level of care is incredible. And his level of passion seeps through. It's clear he is a strong advocate for palliative care and assisted dying hits close to home. And it's something he doesn't want in his home.

The issues surrounding assisted dying really do draw people off the back benches. Often people who would not engage in this level of intensity are all-in. And the rest of us, the silent majority, sit and watch. Like many things in life, we don't want to engage if it doesn't directly affect us. We tend to shy away from taking sides, especially if it is heated.

Personally, I usually eject from thinking when a topic gets too complicated, or if I have no place to put thoughts in. But in this case, I simply can't. The responsibility of the vote on a life-and-death issue carries too much weight to ignore. And the recurring message that this is a 'massive decision' is only reinforcing my need to pursue answers and draw conclusions.

CHAPTER 9:

PROFESSOR MARGARET SOMERVILLE

That's twice now I've met my interviewees in their pyjamas. Professor Margaret Somerville woke to my FaceTime call and answered it. "Oh sorry, I'm still in bed. Usually my cat wakes me but he obviously didn't this morning." We laugh. She's brave answering a video call with a morning face.

Thirty minutes later and Margaret, who goes by Margo, walks me to her lounge in Perth while talking a mile a minute. She wants to know about what journalism I had been involved in. When she worked as a lawyer in Sydney a long time ago Fairfax Media was one of the firm's main clients. She also currently has a boyfriend who is a journalist. Aboriginal art lines the wall and her Bengal cat makes an entrance.

Margo has her reading glasses resting on top of her head and is chipper. I don't have to even ask her a question and we are off racing at full throttle. I'm working hard to keep up. "The decision about whether or not to legalise euthanasia is the single most important values decision of the 21st century."

Really?

"My current work is to try and show people why that's the case. It's a decision about whether we will intentionally kill each other," Margo says. "The foundational value of every civilised society is the value of respect for human life. This value has to be upheld at two levels—the level of each individual life and the level of society in general. Even if

> **"The decision about whether or not to legalise euthanasia is the single most important values decision of the 21st century."**

you could say assisted dying does not breach the value of respect for human life for the individual level, the value of respect at the societal level is definitely breached. And that is so dangerous."

The first pause.

Those are some big statements. I ask for a bit of background on Margo's career and experience to understand what this opinion is founded on.

Margo has got quite the life story. But to stay on track I'll try and summarise her expertise… She has nine doctorates. Graduating from the University of Adelaide with a bachelor in pharmacy, Margo went on to study law at Sydney University. Margo and her former husband moved to Montreal where she gained a PhD in medical law. She went on to tutor at the law faculty of MacGill University Montreal and was offered a job as assistant professor. The Medical Research Council in Canada requested her to join a special committee which was investigating euthanasia and the protection of life. That's when she was thrust into this issue and became a commentator and reviewer appearing on a number of media programmes including a regular radio show. She has authored many books and has had many more academic articles published in journals across the world.

Technically Margo is a bioethicist. And boy, can she talk!

"The pro-euthanasia case is very easy to present—have a horrible story about someone's natural death, and how they were not properly looked after, have terrible pain and suffering. Convert the mystery of death to the problem of death. Because postmodern societies are secular and not religious, they can't deal with the mystery, so it terrorises them. There's a free-floating anxiety of death. So introduce the fact you can choose how you can die. The New Zealand legislation is an absolute extreme paradigm of that. I couldn't believe it when I read that you have a list of choices of how you want to be killed."

What do you think about those who say—'Well it's OK you feel that way but I want to choose this'?

"The base ideology behind this is the respect to the right of an individual's autonomy. Well that's just not true—you're also a member of a family, community and society. Feminists call this 'relational autonomy'; really it's an articulation of 'no man is an island'. It's compared to the intense or radical autonomy which just focuses on the individual. You need to consider the damage you afflict onto relational autonomy."

Having someone who specialises in how to consider medical ethical dilemmas is helpful in this task. Her perspective can be incredibly helpful in understanding context. I ask what Margo thinks about the importance of autonomy in this debate.

"When people say 'I'll take control of this and I'll choose how I die', it's just on an individual person and just in the present. It doesn't look to human memory, to history, of what happens to a society when this is legal. It also doesn't use collective human imagination which says what happens in the future, the potential, the fallout, the consequences."

So you can't make a wise decision without considering the past and the future?

"Exactly. Some of those that have the best handle of looking to the past, present and future, looking to the individual and to the society, are first nations people groups. In Australia and Canada the indigenous people are not promoting this, and are generally completely anti-euthanasia."

Margo says the discussion around assisted dying is essentially a social values/political issue. "Society has to work out whether it wants this or not. But in order to make a wise decision they have to understand the full implications of what they're doing. The problem is by reducing it

> **"We have to ask why for at least 2,000 years have we prohibited doctors from killing people. Why suddenly are we saying now it is alright? Why are we getting doctors to do it?"**

to looking at an individual person, or not looking at the past or future, wise decisions are not being made.

"We have to ask why for at least 2,000 years have we prohibited doctors from killing people. Why suddenly are we saying now it is alright? Why are we getting doctors to do it? Doctors are no more able to answer the question than any other person."

Is this why not all medical practitioners are in 100 per cent agreement about this?

"Yes—although around 92 per cent of palliative care specialists are anti-euthanasia and the literature on it shows definitively palliative care and euthanasia are incompatible and radically opposed."

Obviously the medical field will be the most directly impacted by this law, though, and the majority don't want it. So with historical context can you tell me why this law is so important to the medical field?

"Because doctors have been bound to the Hippocratic Oath for 2,500 years."

The Hippocratic Oath is the earliest expression of medical ethics in the Western world. Originally written by Greek physician Hippocrates in around 470BC it's an oath of ethics historically taken by physicians. It's the equivalent of ethical malpractice to break it. "In ancient societies before modern medicine there were witch doctors. The witch doctor was the person who tried to help you and cure you [the doctor element], and if you had an enemy and wanted them to drop dead, the witch aspect was available. What the Hippocratic Oath did was split apart those two roles of the doctor. The doctor became the healer not the killer.

"What euthanasia does is put the killer back in. That's why it's wrong. The Hippocratic Oath said, 'We will cure where possible, we will care always and we will never kill.' Now we are saying, 'We will cure where we can, we will care always, but we will kill if you want us to.'"

Margo says people want to put the white coat of medicine on assisted dying to legitimise it. "What are our normal assumptions with this white coat? When people see a doctor they expect them to be ethical, to try and help them live as long as possible, because we always think of medical treatment as being at least the intention of doing good and never to do harm. If you put a white cloak on it everyone will think it's OK."

"When people see a doctor they expect them to be ethical, to try and help them live as long as possible, because we always think of medical treatment as being at least the intention of doing good and never to do harm."

She says this would change the medical profession forever... and what sort of society will we be creating if we introduce it? I wonder, if this is a societal issue, then isn't it good we are involving everyone to vote on it in the referendum?

"Something to consider is the fundamental assumption that if a majority votes for something, it means it's ethical. That's wrong. If that were the case, then the Nazi regime in Germany was ethical. The majority of Germans voted for it. I know everyone freaks out when you bring up the Nazi argument. But I've looked into the legislation they introduced on euthanasia and it is similar. Even the way they introduced it was similar."

So, of course, I found an article in the *New York Times* published on 8 October, 1933 entitled 'Nazis plan to kill incurables to end pain; German religious groups oppose move'.

This is what is published (emphasis mine):

> *"Berlin, Oct 7 — The Ministry of Justice in a detailed memorandum explaining the Nazi aims regarding the German penal code today announced its intention to authorise physicians to end the sufferings of incurable patients. The memorandum, still lacking the force of law, proposed that 'it shall be made possible for physicians to end the tortures of incurable patients, upon request, in the interests of true humanity'.*
>
> *The proposed legal recognition of euthanasia—the act of providing a painless and peaceful death—raised a number of fundamental problems of a religious, scientific and legal nature... In medical circles the question was raised as to just when a man is incurable and when his life should be ended.*
>
> *According to the present plans of the Ministry of Justice, incurability would be determined not only by the attending physician, but also by two official doctors who carefully trace the history of the case and personally examine the patient. In insisting that euthanasia shall be permissible only if the accredited attending physician is backed by two experts who so advise, the Ministry believes a guarantee is given that no life still valuable to the state will be wantonly destroyed. The legal question of who may request the application of euthanasia has not been definitely solved. The Ministry merely has proposed that either the patient himself shall 'expressly and earnestly' ask it, or 'in case a patient is no longer able to express his desire, his nearer relatives, acting from motives that do not contravene morals, so request'."*

Margo suggests to note some of the specific wording chosen. The process of safeguards is also included. But everyone knows where that led to.

The New York Times.

Copyright, 1933, by The New York Times Company.

Second-Class Matter, New York, N. Y. NEW YORK, SUNDAY, OCTOBER 8, 1933. F Including Rotogravure Picture, Magazine and Book Sections.

Nazis Plan to Kill Incurables to End Pain; German Religious Groups Oppose Move

By The Associated Press.

BERLIN, Oct. 7.—The Ministry of Justice in a detailed memorandum explaining the Nazi aims regarding the German penal code today announced its intention to authorize physicians to end the sufferings of incurable patients.

The memorandum, still lacking the force of law, proposed that "it shall be made possible for physicians to end the tortures of incurable patients, upon request, in the interests of true humanity."

This proposed legal recognition of euthanasia—the act of providing a painless and peaceful death—raised a number of fundamental problems of a religious, scientific and legal nature.

The Catholic newspaper Germania hastened to observe:

"The Catholic faith binds the conscience of its followers not to accept this method of shortening the sufferings of incurables who are tormented by pain."

In Lutheran circles, too, life is regarded as something that God alone can take.

A large section of the German people, it was expected in some interested circles, might ignore the provisions for euthanasia, which overnight has become a widely-discussed word in the Reich.

In medical circles the question was raised as to just when a man is incurable and when his life should be ended.

According to the present plans of the Ministry of Justice, incurability would be determined not only by the attending physician, but also by two official doctors who would carefully trace the history of the case and personally examine the patient.

In insisting that euthanasia shall be permissible only if the accredited attending physician is backed by two experts who so advise, the Ministry believes a guarantee is given that no life still valuable to the State will be wantonly destroyed.

The legal question of who may request the application of euthanasia has not been definitely solved. The Ministry merely has proposed that either the patient himself shall "expressly and earnestly" ask it, or "in case the patient no longer is able to express his desire, his nearer relatives, acting from motives that do not contravene morals, so request."

"I'm scared we don't know what we are doing... How enormously serious this is. We have to ask ourselves, 'Why now? Why now are we thinking euthanasia is a good idea?' It's not like we have new technology to kill people. We've got excellent pain and suffering treatment… I think it's because of broad societal reasons which include existential factors, loss of hope, loss of meaning, loss of the sense of there being something special about being a human."

Margo says she doesn't mean those who want to use it are hopeless cases. But rather, they have lost hope—most often lost because their hope was dependent on having a connection to the future. "People who are dying haven't got a long-term future, but it doesn't mean you don't have something to look forward to. Even someone coming to visit, or something like music in their palliative care unit… that brings hope."

She says we have to stop regarding hope as a passive thing. "You can actually make hope. You can make it for people. That's what we have got to do."

"You can actually make hope. You can make it for people. That's what we have got to do."

Margo says we should look at the life of famous writer Viktor Frankl. He was in the Auschwitz concentration camp. "After he survived he was interviewed and asked, 'How did you help people?' He said, 'If you give people a why to live, they can find a how to live.' What's missing is the 'why' to live."

Creating hope could change the choice of some suffering in the face of death, but what about those who are adamant about what they want—don't we need to respect their autonomy?

Margo says that under the premise of autonomy, safeguards of protection will not hold. And the law will have to change its eligibility criteria. "Once you understand the main argument—the right of radical autonomy—you will see where the logic progresses. What initially started off as strict safeguards very quickly became modified. In the Netherlands, originally you had to be mentally competent, give an informed decision and suffer irremediably. They argued, 'What about the people who aren't competent and yet are suffering—how can we not allow them the same right?'

"So they changed its interpretation to allow them to have access—someone can give an advance directive if their illness will impact their competence in the future.

"In Canada the legislation is four years old and when it was first introduced it was only for a competent adult who is terminal, in unrelievable suffering, and gives informed decision at the time of euthanasia. They currently are in courts dropping the terminal illness factor, they're looking at allowing advance directives—so you can write a 'living will' to request it, and they are looking at euthanasia for children. There has already been an article published by a group of paediatricians saying the biggest children's hospital in Canada would be willing to provide it if it were legalised."

"There has already been an article published by a group of paediatricians saying the biggest children's hospital in Canada would be willing to provide it if it were legalised."

She says the premise of autonomy, if followed through, will continue to widen. New Zealand's law will not be exempt. "The longest experiment, the Netherlands and Belgium, has shown euthanasia becomes normalised."

Margo has just finished writing a foreword in a book made up of a collection of essays by doctors and nurses in Belgium and their experiences of euthanasia. She has studied the nations and their changes with the assisted dying laws for 40 years.

"This book documents how traumatic euthanasia can be—not just for the family, but also for doctors and nurses. One in 20 nurses and doctors are traumatised by this. They develop mental health problems. The same is happening to family members who are present when they observe euthanasia."

Margo says those close to her have been traumatised by it too. "I was in Canada recently and a friend's partner had just been euthanised. He was a doctor and had found out he had terminal cancer. He asked one of his friends from the hospital to come to his house and euthanise him. My friend and I were sitting in a French bistro in Montreal and suddenly she burst into these uncontrollable sobs and kept saying, 'Margo, it was horrible, it was horrible'.

"People think by providing euthanasia we will remove the trauma and pain and suffering of the person dying and family that have to watch it. But cases out of the Netherlands and Belgium show by trying to prevent trauma, we are causing it. It never just affects the person using it." We have to ask ourselves if this is where we want to go, Margo says.

"People think by providing euthanasia we will remove the trauma and pain and suffering of the person dying and family that have to watch it. But cases out of the Netherlands and Belgium show by trying to prevent trauma, we are causing it. It never just affects the person using it."

She has just finished writing an essay titled *Could the wonder equation help us be more ethical?*.

"I've made an equation—Amazement, wonder and awe plus scepticism (minus nihilism and cynicism) can elicit gratitude and hope, which equates to ethics. I propose that individual and collective experiences of 'amazement, wonder and awe' have the power to enrich our lives, help us to find meaning, bridge the secular/religious divide, and change how we see the world."

A poetic reflection...

My life, my choice
Have you ever been in love?
Love changes life from me to we
From I to us
Once was mine, but now is ours

The beauty of connection
Sharing soul and heart
Alone no longer
Together forever
Only in death will we part

But until that day arrives
I cling to your hand
And carry you through
For a sorrow shared, is a sorrow-halved.

CHAPTER 10:

DR JACK HAVILL

Dr Jack Havill's formidable voice is equipped with 30 years of experience as an intensive care medicine specialist. Now retired, he's the co-author of book *Dying Badly*, organiser of the Doctors Say Yes letter and former president of the End-of-Life Choice Society. He has a down-to-Earth demeanour and doesn't mind sporting a loud 1980s retro jumper while at his home in Hamilton. It certainly keeps me alert for the duration of our Skype call.

Why is Jack so invested in this law change?

After years working in intensive care he eventually wondered if, at times, keeping people alive was actually helping them. "I'd regularly see a person being taken off the respirator and it would result in their death. We called it passive euthanasia, but you were actually doing something that caused death. Usually it would be done after talking to their family if the patient wasn't well enough to consent. Sometimes it was the patient themselves requesting it. It all started my thinking."

That, and the thought of possibly living with the likes of severe dementia, would be intolerable to Jack. "If I couldn't recognise my family and was incontinent, and had to be helped out of bed… I wouldn't want anybody to resuscitate me. I'd like to have the option of an advance directive for assisted dying… to ask, 'When I reach this stage could you please help me die?'."

That advance directive isn't included in the EOLC Act, but it is written into a number of equivalent laws internationally. "The withdrawal of care is an active thing. People talk negatively about assisted dying being an active thing you want from the doctor. But it's not that different... A lot of the concepts aren't new."

Jack says withdrawing treatment and assisted dying are both done to relieve suffering. "No one wants to kill or murder anybody, it's just what you do to help."

"If I couldn't recognise my family and was incontinent, and had to be helped out of bed... I wouldn't want anybody to resuscitate me. I'd like to have the option of an advance directive for assisted dying... to ask, 'When I reach this stage could you please help me die?'."

That's something Jack says palliative care specialists struggle with, always claiming they never intend to kill, and always promising to help relieve suffering. "But there's a group of people whose suffering can't be relieved. Even with palliative sedation, all they are doing is pretending they are helping the patient and family in their suffering. The family just sits there for a week or two while the patient is slowly dying.

"There's also many people who don't get sedation and suffer from a lot of other things, not just pain. Things like the indignity of incontinence, hallucinations, going in and out of consciousness. It can be a traumatic time and family are just sitting there wishing it were the end. What's the use of that?"

Jack says it's because palliative care was developed largely by the Catholic Church that it has a fixation against assisted dying. "In Australia the majority of hospices are run by Catholics. The Catholic hierarchy has decreed they should never allow someone to die. It's all to do with God deciding when you die: you are His, it's His life. But the thing is we have already taken that control from God when we provide treatment."

It's hypocritical to elongate life for one but refuse to end it for another, says Jack. "Aren't both playing God?"

While many palliative care providers are refusing involvement in other jurisdictions, some are changing. "In countries like Belgium and the Netherlands, which are Catholic based, they are starting to say they will work together to provide it. In Canada some Catholic people say they won't attend an assisted death, but others will. While there is a strong lobby from the palliative hierarchy against assisted dying in New Zealand there are plenty of nurses in support of it."

It's that alternative perspective Jack wanted to raise when he presented the Doctors Say Yes letter.

"The Doctors Say No campaign was putting big advertisements in the newspapers with a whole list of names. They had 1,500 names and were claiming they represented doctors. We have 30 doctors in our group and we thought we would just put the opposing view in."

"No one wants to kill or murder anybody, it's just what you do to help."

Jack says he is confident a lot of doctors will come on board if the Act is passed. "At the end of the day, there's going to be a need for a pool of doctors willing to participate if this law passes. I think there will be. There could be some difficulties to get enough doctors in rural areas, though. Some opponents complain, saying there will only be a few doctors doing all of the work… Well whose fault is that?!"

The EOLC Act says doctors are not allowed to initiate a conversation about assisted dying but Jack says that condition is "stupid". "When you are talking to a patient you want to discuss all their options. People just put that in the law because they are worried about doctors pressuring patients. But the last thing a doctor wants to do is help a patient die."

Jack says hinging a law change on a referendum is a bad decision. "Very few people understand the ramifications of it, whether they are for it or opposed to it. We have always said it needs to be decided by a group of intelligent people who have worked through all the issues. This referendum is a waste of money. The one good thing is at least the groundwork has been done on the Act and it will be passed if it gets the votes."

Another beef Jack has with the Act is the criteria of the six-month prognosis.

"There's a group of patients that are suffering immensely, like those with motor neuron disease, where they get weaker and weaker and might go on for a few years. They don't meet the criteria and are the sorts of people who will continue to commit suicide."

"There's a group of patients that are suffering immensely, like those with motor neuron disease, where they get weaker and weaker and might go on for a few years. They don't meet the criteria and are the sorts of people who will continue to commit suicide."

He says while the opponents are always talking about how this will encourage suicide, those in favour of the law are trying to discourage it.

But isn't there a very clear similarity between assisted dying and 'normal' suicide?

Jack says no. "There is confusion in terminology. Suicide is done usually by a mentally unstable person. Almost all suicides are done by irrational people, and they happen quickly without other people's involvement. They cause a lot of heartache and grief to the remaining family."

He says they are done by people who could have had the option of living on if they went to the right places to get support. "Assisted dying is different because you are actually a rational person. You're going to die anyway. Although you may not die for several years, or in this law, for six months, you just want to avoid suffering. So you consult medical practitioners.

"At the moment there's quite a significant group of terminally-ill patients who commit suicide. That is awful. That's one thing we hope will stop. Those cases are what I call 'rational suicide'."

"At the moment there's quite a significant group of terminally-ill patients who commit suicide. That is awful. That's one thing we hope will stop. Those cases are what I call 'rational suicide'."

How will the EOLC Act weed out 'suicidal' people from those who should have access to assisted dying?

"Patients will have to have discussions with the doctor. The doctor can pick up any mental instability. Any person can do that. If we talk to someone and ask, 'Why do they want to do it?'—you would soon pick up the person was not right."

Jack says people also worry about families pressuring patients to seek assisted dying so they can gain inheritance. "But it doesn't take much to detect that. I don't think this has been a real issue, and it hasn't been an issue overseas."

I rebut that comment with the fact that Oregon's annual assisted dying reports show people regularly list 'feeling like a burden on family' as a reason to apply for assisted suicide.

"The person can be there suffering enormously themselves and then feeling like their family members should be off with their kids.

It's part of the suffering that happens. It's not unreasonable to feel like a burden. Old people feel a burden to their children... Sometimes children feel a burden to their mother. I'd be surprised if not everybody feels a burden to someone when they are going through suffering. I don't think that's a reason to oppose it. You can ask the question if they are a real burden, and are dying anyway, and have suffering—why shouldn't that be a reason why they also ask for assisted dying? It might not be a family intentionally doing it, but it's part of the suffering."

So when you get down to it, it's really just offering people the choice?

"You're not even offering people a choice... You're giving people the option of the choice. You're not going out there saying, 'You should do this,' but just making it possible for a person to take this route."

I wonder how Jack reconciles the potential for error if it really all comes down to just offering an option.

"You've got to look at the bigger picture. Let's say somehow someone slides through the cracks; I don't know how it would happen, but just suppose they would have lived for three years instead of six months... Why should you disadvantage all those other people for the sake of a very occasional thing that goes wrong?"

"How safe do we say a law has to be before we are comfortable with saying it's good?"

Jack says if we applied that theory to cardiac surgery, which is high-risk, we wouldn't be operating on hearts at all. "How safe do we say a law has to be before we are comfortable with saying it's good?," he asks.

In fact, this law will help make it more safe considering there is research showing around 4.5 per cent of doctors are already 'knocking people off', Jack says.

He is referring to a study conducted in 2013 by a group of three University of Auckland professors, including Associate Professor

Phillipa Malpas, who was a member of the Voluntary Euthanasia Society. The study was done to explore medical decision-making practices at the end-of-life made by GPs in New Zealand. A postal questionnaire was sent to 3,420 GPs and anonymous phone interviews were also made. A total of 650 GPs responded (21 per cent), and of these, 359 (65.5 per cent) reported making an end-of-life medical decision. Of those, 4.5 per cent attributed death to a drug that had been prescribed, supplied or administered explicitly for the purpose of hastening the patient's death.

"The EOLC Act isn't what we wanted particularly; it doesn't go far enough. We would like for it to include people who are suffering but are not at their end-of-life, and advance directives so people with dementia would be eligible."

Yet I question whether legalising something because it already happens is the right response to law-breakers.

I ask Jack what the plan is if the law does not pass the referendum.

"We will just keep trying. This will happen eventually… it's a tide which is flowing across the world. The EOLC Act isn't what we wanted particularly; it doesn't go far enough. We would like for it to include people who are suffering but are not at their end-of-life, and advance directives so people with dementia would be eligible."

I've heard a lot of people talk about a 'bad death' experience surrounding the loss of a loved one. But I can't help thinking about how similar this practice is to that of people sharing their birthing stories.

When I was pregnant with my first child I became acutely aware of the potential for pain and the risks to my own health and that of my baby's. Horror stories seemed to come from every corner. Did anyone have a positive birth story? I had to decide early on to monitor the amount of people I spoke to about it.

Science has shown that the presence of fear in the midst of a birth has a tremendous effect on your brain's ability to release hormones that relax your body and help it along the labour process. The last thing I needed was to be up at night worrying about the impending birth.

I can't help but wonder what the impact of negative death stories and experiences have on us. Many of us are carrying grief, unanswered questions, disappointments and trauma from those experiences. And there is both little education given before a person dies, and very little support offered afterwards.

But, I mean, it happens to everyone—surely we should just 'get on with life'?

Seeing the pain and anguish so many MPs have shared during their speeches in Parliament through the three readings of this legislation has proven to me we haven't adequately dealt with it. Tears are an indication that pain is still present. And we can't just 'move on'; we need to talk about it... get proper help and healing.

Postnatal depression is very common in New Zealand among mothers in the months after they give birth. A lot of research into the causes and tendencies has been done. One of the potential triggers includes having a traumatic birth experience. If trauma happens in birth, surely it happens in death too.

In New Zealand, when you are pregnant you are invited and encouraged to attend a 'antenatal course' near the end of your pregnancy to prepare you for labour and birth. Parent Centres across the country provide the service as well as hospitals and district health boards. Thousands of Kiwi mums and dads are thrust into activities and conversations around a table of complete strangers about things you normally wouldn't get caught dead talking about.

In our first week we were told to draw a diagram of a woman's body and label the working parts involved in birth... including a vagina, uterus, cervix... The young men and women both had to work together to draw and locate each part. And there were plenty of red faces and awkward moments we now laugh about.

Led by an educator we went on a journey of discovering what to expect, what is 'normal', the nutrients scientists have found in breast milk, and the side effects of birth intervention, such as how epidurals can affect a baby. It was fact based with the intention to inform, not to judge or rate someone's birth journey. The course was one of the most critically important times for me personally in preparing to give birth and walk through the biggest 'marathon' I'd ever signed up for.

Why do we not find a way to educate people about death to the same degree? Science can be incredibly helpful to dispel fears and debunk myths around the process of death.

The medical industry is a world of its own—and I know for myself that being introduced to systems and protocols during the last moments of my granddad's life was not the best time to be thrown into it.

Every single one of us will face death. And the fear of the unknown is a real thing. Could this fear be influencing our decision as to whether assisted dying is the right way forward?

---

CHAPTER 11:

DR HUHANA HICKEY MNZM

"Personal Account

If there's anyone who could talk about looking death at the face, it would be Dr Huhana Hickey.

It feels like Huhana has lived five lives in one. She's survived three suicide attempts, been in several comas. She's had bouts with depression, cancer and has a rare form of multiple sclerosis. Trauma seemed to knock on her door before she was born. Yet her story is one of embracing life and overcoming fear. I talk to her while her wheelchair is parked at her kitchen bench.

It's a week after Huhana's had surgery to remove a renal tumour. She's recovering reasonably quickly and thankfully the growth was found to be benign.

Halfway through our interview she needs to duck out to the bathroom and discusses the difficulty of using a catheter for the first time. Huhana isn't one to hide anything. She says it like it is.

And it's her different perspective that I appreciate. I guess her multiple brushes with death have forced her to stare some serious life issues in the face and not cower from them. That, and the fact she is a lawyer, a Member of the New Zealand Order of Merit, has a PhD in philosophy and, among other things, has been an advisor for the

Ministry of Social Development and a panel member for the Human Rights Review Committee.

Huhana's styling a sort of mohawk with her short dark hair. She's feisty, direct... her persona a little dark even. But under that all, you can see compassion, hope and a disposition of gratitude towards life.

There's been a history of genocide and eugenics (a movement that is aimed at improving the genetic composition of the human race, often achieved by selective breeding) in every ancestral line Huhana has. "As an indigenous person, my Ngarigo [Australian Aboriginal] ancestors were given smallpox blankets to kill them. Sugar and tobacco were given to both the Māori and Aborigines, and the Sami population were almost eradicated completely in Norway and Finland. All of those are in my ancestral lines, so I've lived the history of eugenics and colonisation and attempts of genocide."

"The death of six million Jews all began with disabled people being targeted first. Once it was perfected on the disabled they extended it to the gays, the gypsies and to the Jews. I'm surprised people don't realise how much hatred towards the disabled exists historically."

If that wasn't enough, Huhana says there is massive discrimination in the area of disability. "The death of six million Jews all began with disabled people being targeted first. Once it was perfected on the disabled they extended it to the gays, the gypsies and to the Jews. I'm surprised people don't realise how much hatred towards the disabled exists historically."

I catch myself doing some introspection on my own knowledge

surrounding historical discrimination around disabled people… I come up pretty short.

"The Greeks did it, Aristotle talked about it, the Spartans wiped themselves out of existence looking for perfection."

Huhana says we are still attempting perfection. "We place value on perfection, but we are not placing value on imperfection. And that's part of the problem. Until we address society's attitudes how can we say this Act will be fair and equal? That it will provide a better society? It's got nothing to do with easing the pain of people's suffering. Euthanasia is about privilege of choice. The argument is it's a way to alleviate pain—the concept of having control brings peace.

"Introducing law like this is not going to eradicate suffering."

"It's affluent Western countries seeking to euthanise people. Indigenous peoples aren't doing it. It's predominantly white people wanting to have control of their lives.

"Look, I'm pro-choice, but under the Crimes Act if you want to end your life, you are completely able to. To me it's cowardly asking someone else to do it for you."

She says legislating on the basis of a subjective issue like pain and suffering can't be done. "Introducing law like this is not going to eradicate suffering."

Huhana says it is dangerous giving someone the legal right to kill you. "Once you have given that power to another person they can coerce you or pressure you into it. And sometimes people will be given assisted dying when all they really needed was help to live."

That power handed over to doctors is even more dangerous considering they have little understanding of what it is like to live with a disability.

"Doctors often don't know our unique needs. We are all different because we happen to all be humans. We all present differently. We are not a textbook and that's why you can't apply a textbook answer."

She says it isn't just doctors who don't understand. "Society labels, marginalises, compartmentalises and places us in positions. I can't really blame people who don't understand—I had never seen a disabled person myself until I met a refugee who survived polio when I was in high school. Back in the '80s they used to put them [disabled people] in residential care and wouldn't bring them out into the community.

"We say this is all about someone's choice, but disabled people often aren't given good choices around healthcare at all and the sector is majorly underfunded."

"Society's attitudes towards disabled people still is one of wanting us excluded and not included. The younger generation don't have an understanding of history, and they don't know why we have our concerns."

Huhana says facts prove her point—disabled people die at a much higher rate than everybody else in residential care. They are often not proactively resuscitated. And they are extremely reliant on the care and support they receive from others to live a full life. This reliance on support, often funded by the Government, puts disabled people in a very difficult situation when something like assisted dying is introduced, Huhana says.

"We say this is all about someone's choice, but disabled people often aren't given good choices around healthcare at all and the sector is majorly underfunded. We have to ask ourselves whether the move for assisted dying law is economically tied. Our health system is at breaking point financially—half a billion in debt over disability funding alone.

"How much are we influenced by the issue of pain, or being a burden, or how much are we really influenced by economics and not being able to provide essential services to people? Until we address issues around funding of disability and palliative care there is no such thing as choice. This Act is full of risks."

From a legal perspective Huhana says this Act hasn't properly been risk-protected. "The amendments suggested in the SOPs [Supplementary Order Papers] were designed to mitigate the risks but they were all voted down, which astonished the sh*t out of me. We've basically got a law geared towards a small part of our population that will actually aim at a larger group."

Huhana says she was shocked to read a comment on MP Carmel Sepuloni's Facebook page from a mother begging for the Bill to be legalised so she could have her severely disabled daughter euthanised. "Don't tell me we are safe when we have parents, partners and others who are actively wanting to end our lives."

Huhana says she was shocked to read a comment on MP Carmel Sepuloni's Facebook page from a mother begging for the Bill to be legalised so she could have her severely disabled daughter euthanised. "Don't tell me we are safe when we have parents, partners and others who are actively wanting to end our lives."

The intensity has been dialled up in our conversation and the direction has landed us in a few fringe areas. I want to know more about what Huhana thinks is the right way forward if assisted dying is the wrong one.

"Dying a good death comes down to attitude and how to address your fear. When I work with people who are dying I sit with them; I don't care how long it takes. I listen to their fear and we talk through it. In Māoridom I'm seen as matakite, which means I can see the other side. For Māori I'm able to talk to them about their ancestors. The fear goes. About a month later they pass away and they all pass away well, because they faced the fear. It's nothing to be afraid of, but people are frightened. We have to talk about it.

"The best way to combat fear is face it. Face the fear that's going on. But the problem is we are now legislating a way out. We're pandering to people's fear. You won't be afraid. You won't be in pain or suffering. But you will be dead.

"I'm alive today when I'm not meant to be, I don't know how long I've got but I focus on that. If you focus on that you're not living your life. One of the keys to break through the fear is to live each day as though it is your last.

"I'm not afraid to die. If it comes to me I'm ready. But if I push myself to die I'm taking away times with my grandchildren, my partner, my family. I'm in quite a bit of pain but it's life. I try and ride through the pain. I try to understand what it's for. It's there to teach us, to guide us. If it's too much you take more pain relief and you get through that day because the next day can be easier."

Is the pain and suffering worth it?

"Well, I haven't got a choice. There's things I wanted to do, dreams I had… I'm losing the use of my hand and I've been a cartoonist. My voice is going and I love to sing. The things I love I'm losing the ability to do myself. But I can listen to my favourite singers and I can look at my favourite artists. I enjoy watching students evolve ideas. I'm asking who do I mentor, who do I support, who can I help through a journey of their own. I've got a responsibility there. If I let myself down I let them down.

"My grandson just sees his nanna. He lives in Sydney so they video-call me. He blows kisses to me in his videos; there's unconditional love.

"Life is more than pain, suffering, disability, emotions or fears. Life is when you wake up in the morning and take your first breath and it's silent; it's the very first moment of contemplation. You have the curtains open and can see the red-tipped dawn rising and you think, 'Ah, red in the morning, shepherd's warning'. Each day is different to the day before. The pain from yesterday is not the pain today. Every day is good. You've got to change your attitude, your mindset. Mine used to be glass half empty. Now it is half full. And if it looks like it is emptying then look for a way to fill it. Whatever it is that moves you. I'm a zombie freak. If I'm feeling angry I go watch a zombie movie. Something you enjoy, something quirky.

"People focus on their fear so much they don't look around them. They don't know how to address it. To them they think euthanasia is: take a pill, get an injection and it's over. They don't look past that and realise they will never wake up again."

I ask her if she wants to die.

"To be honest, I wouldn't mind dying. But then I see a photo of my grandchild and it gives me joy. I know what my future holds and know it won't be easy. But there's things that help to make it bearable and doable. If I sit in my own anxiety and fear, I won't have a life.

"People focus on their fear so much they don't look around them. They don't know how to address it. To them they think euthanasia is: take a pill, get an injection and it's over. They don't look past that and realise they will never wake up again."

"For me my life has not been easy. I've had to fight from the minute I was born and I've constantly had to fight. I learnt I had to fight for other people as well. What people don't realise is everyone has a struggle in their life. Everyone experiences pain. It's about finding yourself and understanding where you stand in this world—that's the key.

"We all die. They might think they are controlling it… but accidents happen every day. People don't plan to be disabled or get sick. No one plans it. It's part of being human."

It's by observing people dying that Huhana's beliefs have been solidified. "I had to watch it to understand."

She has watched several people die by assisted suicide on YouTube for exploratory purposes. "I watched a video of a young Dutch woman who had been given a diagnosis and decided it was her time to go. She could still walk and do everything; she looked relatively healthy and well.

"The woman had two friends with her when the doctor came to give her the legal dose of medication. It was just like a normal doctor's appointment. Everything was very clinical. It didn't feel spiritual or nice at all.

"The woman had chosen the clothes she wanted to wear and had everything laid out ready. She was talking to her friends when the doctor asked, "Is this what you want? The woman said, 'Yes'. Then the doctor prepared the solution, and said, 'Again, I must ask you—is this what you want?' The woman agreed a second time. The doctor put the medication in a glass and with juice. She drank it down and all her friends were talking and laughing and drinking cups of tea.

"The woman sat back on the couch, which was covered in plastic (because people lose control of their body functions as they die), eating a bit of chocolate, which is what they offer people because the drugs are bitter.

"The doctor took her vitals as she was talking. Then the woman started slurring her speech. The doctor said, 'You're going to go to sleep now.' So the woman closed her eyes… and she was gone. You could hear her friends say, 'That's it?'. And the doctor replied, 'That's it. It's over now.'"

Huhana said it struck her as cold, clinical and sanitised. "Are we going to do that to death now? We are not going to have that beautiful experience anymore."

It's in stark contrast to other stories Huhana has of walking with families and friends to the end.

"I had a friend who was given one month to live… she had lung cancer. She was married to a Fijian Indian and had two young lads. We got the extended family over and they took over the process; we put her in the lounge on a bed. When I talked to her at the beginning she was scared. Every day we made a video for her youngest son, so he would never forget his mum.

"She eventually ended up in a coma. On the day she died we had moved her back into the bedroom… I was sitting there with her in my arms and she opened her eyes, looked at me and said, 'Thank you'." Huhana says she closed her eyes and passed away.

"How can people choosing assisted dying not leave trauma? It becomes all about the individual but not about the family that stays behind."

"There's a reason why. A reason why we should leave this process. Death is a normal part of life. It is painful. But it is time to say goodbye. How can people choosing assisted dying not leave trauma? It becomes all about the individual but not about the family that stays behind. How do they reconcile between death and dying? It's an unfinished business act.

"It just ends a life, but it doesn't conclude anything."

As hard as it may be observing someone's decline into death, I can't help wondering if part of the beauty is in the process of saying goodbye.

The quick and immediate death of a person choosing assisted dying feels much more like a 'see you later' process. Not the finality and slow process of really shutting down to the world, the circle of closeness getting smaller—the reality of forever leaving and releasing is cut short abruptly.

Sure, I know people hold 'death parties' as a sort of pre-funeral, and people say they feel as though they get the control of a healthy farewell on their own terms. But something just doesn't sit right.

Reading stories of those overseas who have chosen death on their own terms through assisted dying has not brought me a respect but rather a sadness or sense of cheapening the experience.

Unfortunately, staring at death in the face and no longer running from it in denial will confront some things we otherwise wouldn't normally allow.

I recall a Canadian doctor telling a story about a patient she helped euthanise… they had requested Frank Sinatra's *I Did it My Way* for their final moment. The story still burns in my memory and leaves a sick feeling in my stomach. The song choice felt like an ultimate act of defiance.

In my time of reflecting I read an excerpt from a book by Kiwi author George A.F. Seber called *Coping With Dying*. He wrote: "*A dying person who has found peace and acceptance in their death will have to separate themselves, step by step, from their environment, including their most loved ones. How can a person be ready to die if he or she continues to hold onto meaningful relationships rather than letting go? As an aside, I should mention that we do not need to protect children from the process of dying but we need to allow time for them to say goodbye and emphasise, if needed, that it is not their fault. We need to explain openly and honestly and allow for questions.*"

I catch myself tearing up… the one line that snags my heart: "*How can a person be ready to die if he or she continues to hold on to meaningful relationships rather than letting go?*".

Personally one of my greatest fears is losing someone. Not so much the way they go, but rather it's the darkness on the other side. The grief. The isolation. The abandonment of a loved one. The hole they leave and the pain of a gaping wound of memory. I have to stop and check where this pain comes from.

Immediately I remember back to a difficult time in my teenage years. It has taken me years to process poignant memories from that period. And the pain is still present in a few. The depth of grief at times surfaces and I discover my own coping mechanisms, most of which are about avoidance.

I think we all have moments in time where something has been cut and its scar has not healed properly. Unfortunately, staring at death in the face and no longer running from it in denial will confront some things we otherwise wouldn't normally allow. But these things are important. They can ultimately influence the direction of life we take; what we listen to, or are willing to consider. Denial is a powerful director of thoughts. And courage is needed to confront it.

SECTION 4:

LEGAL THOUGHTS

An ethical dilemma: *A petrol tanker skids and overturns on a lonely inter-state highway in the United States, leaving the driver trapped in his cab. He watches with horror as petrol begins to leak from the tank onto the engine block.*

First on the scene is a highway patrolman. He sees the driver's predicament and knows the rescue services will take far too long to reach such an isolated spot.

"Shoot me," the driver calls out; "I don't want to burn to death." The policeman chose to comply.

Was the policeman right to shoot the driver? It's a difficult question to answer.

Some years ago a parliamentary committee in London which was enquiring into whether assisted dying should be legalised put the question to a range of experts. No one was able to give a clear answer—until one said, "Yes, I would do as the policeman did". Then he added, "but I wouldn't expect the law to be changed to allow that."

"Laws are made for every day. They are not made for exceptional circumstances. But they also contain discretion to deal sensibly with exceptions."
– Robert Preston, UK euthanasia expert

Law to me is like maths. Complicated. And not my natural strong point. So with some trepidation I enter the realm with questions in hand. But it must be done.

The binding referendum we will vote on is all about a piece of law. This one piece of legislation wields enough power to bring death and must provide just as strong a shield to protect life.

The EOLC Act has been contributed to by a lawmaking team, including the late Lecretia Seales. Her husband, Matthew Vickers, has called it "smart, robust and evidence based".

"Lecretia was a law reformer and well respected among the legal community. She worked for two prime ministers: Sir John Key, as a justice advisor, and Sir Geoffrey Palmer QC, as a senior legal advisor at the Law Commission. She knew exactly what she was asking for, and its legal implications, and she would be pleased with the End of Life Choice Bill, which has been crafted with the assistance of lawyers who acted for Lecretia in Seales v Attorney-General," Matthew says. "Those lawyers have been steeped in this issue for years and have a deep understanding of how the laws work overseas. They are this country's legal experts on this issue. And despite misrepresentations from opponents, this Bill stands up as one of the best examples of all of them, tailored to the needs of New Zealanders."

Yet submissions to the Justice Select Committee from lawyers, legal experts and Queen's Counsel members would beg to differ. I knock on the doors of three experts in their fields to see why.

CHAPTER 12:

RICHARD MCLEOD

Richard is giving me a couple of hours to talk through his views on the EOLC Act from his lounge in Ōrākei, Auckland. We just clock week one of COVID-19 level-four lockdown and he, like me, is attempting to work from home with two young children running around.

Richard is a human rights, immigration and refugee lawyer with 25 years experience in his field, and he's leading a group called Lawyers for Vulnerable New Zealanders that are raising their serious concerns about the End of Life Choice Act. The group includes a diverse range of practising lawyers, legal advisors, academics and Queen's Counsel members. Among them are those who support assisted dying in principle, but emphatically oppose this Act.

The resounding concern among them is the threat this "poorly drafted law" poses on vulnerable people in our country. "We are alarmed by what this Act is proposing, so feel we must warn all New Zealanders about the extreme dangers it will pose to our country and our most vulnerable people," Richard says.

Immediately I can see similarities between Richard and David Seymour. They are both quick, intelligent, succinct and dedicated... and around the same age. But they sit on polar ends of this issue. And while both have a form of respect for their counterpart, it's clear neither is particularly fond of each other.

"Our laws are woven together very intricately and delicately to serve the common good. When you start tampering with our most fundamental laws just because it suits your own purposes or, as David claims, 'It's only for a few people', then things really start to unravel."

Richard says that's what the experience with assisted dying regimes around the world shows us. He has studied international euthanasia laws for several years and has dismembered the one that sits before us. One of his conclusions: vulnerable people will be dramatically impacted by it. He's worried Kiwis don't really know what they are voting for.

"If people understood how this law will impact the most vulnerable among us, then poll numbers would change overnight."

"The pro-euthanasia lobby has found ways to dumb down their message to propagandise it for mass consumption. The real issues are being hidden. If people understood how this law will impact the most vulnerable among us, then poll numbers would change overnight. Would you support a law that would make our elderly people feel like they should kill themselves prematurely? One that would allow abusers to manipulate elderly victims into dying early? That is what will happen if this law is adopted."

That's a slamming report which is backed by the group that have identified at least 30 fatal flaws within the Act. The majority of their concerns lie around coercion issues. While I'm not going to list them all, I ask Richard what his greatest concern among them is.

"The potential for coercion of vulnerable people, and the fact there's really nothing in the Act to stop it."

Those in support of assisted dying are adamant the law change is not for vulnerable people. They say vulnerable people aren't the ones opting to use it internationally and they will be protected by safeguards.

But Richard challenges that theory.

"First of all, what is your definition of vulnerable? I've been working with vulnerable people for 25 years so I think I know one when I see one. The New Zealand Human Rights Commission's definition of a vulnerable person is expansive. It includes anybody who is dependent on a carer, or has been diagnosed with a chronic or terminal illness, over 75, or over 65 and living alone, or who lives in severe financial hardship. A person is vulnerable if they are 'less likely than other people to cope and recover from stresses and pressures'. These are the ones using it."

> **"For a country that prides itself on protecting the 'little guy' and on how well we treat our most vulnerable as part of our mantra, we could easily become a country that starts to think it's acceptable for a vulnerable person to end their lives."**

Richard refers to the Oregon Public Health Division's annual Death With Dignity reports which have shown that between 63 and 67 per cent of people in Oregon who chose assisted suicide in the last five years were enrolled with the Oregon Health Plan Medicare or Medicaid insurance schemes. These are state insurance schemes for people on low incomes. He also refers to reports which show anywhere between 25 and 75 per cent of terminal patients suffer from depression at some point in their illness.

"Receiving a terminal prognosis is probably the most vulnerable time a person has had in their entire life. It's a time where people are extremely vulnerable and susceptible to manipulative action, coercion or even suggestion. For a country that prides itself on protecting the 'little guy' and on how well we treat our most vulnerable as part of our mantra, we could easily become a country that starts to think it's acceptable for a vulnerable person to end their lives."

Richard says if there is even just one case of wrongful practice in any jurisdiction using this type of law, then we shouldn't accept it. "And there are more than a handful of cases where this has happened. Abuse of vulnerable people is endemic in these systems."

I ask for examples. "Roger Foley and Candice Lewis." Both cases are from Canada and involve people with severe disabilities being pressured into requesting assisted dying by their doctors or specialists as a solution to their medical problems. The Canadian law, like ours, requires a patient to initiate the conversation about assisted dying with a doctor; the doctor is not allowed to suggest it as a course of action.

Roger Foley launched a lawsuit against a Canadian hospital, several health agencies, the Ontario Government and the Federal Government after he said on two occasions that his doctors were the ones to suggest he choose physician-assisted dying as a solution to the struggle he was having in getting proper self-directed care funding.

CTV News covered the story in 2018 and Roger publicly released audio recordings of the conversations he had with doctors. In one recording Roger is asked how he is doing and if he felt like harming himself. Roger is heard saying he was always thinking he wanted to end his life because of the way he was being treated at the hospital and because his requests for self-directed care were denied. The doctor responded, telling Roger he could "just apply to get an assisted" if he wanted to end his life.

In Candice Lewis' case her mum, Sheila Elson, was offered euthanasia by a doctor in the hallway at a hospital when her 25-year-old daughter had been admitted there with serious pain. Candice had several medical conditions, including spina bifida, cerebral palsy and chronic seizure disorder.

Sheila was told by the doctor her daughter was dying and she was "being selfish" for not considering the treatment. The pair had asked the hospital for an apology but did not take legal action. CBC reported the story in 2017. The hospital had responded by offering to sit down and discuss the issue. Neither Roger nor Candice chose to receive assisted dying.

"Vulnerable people like Candice and Roger must be highly protected, but the Act offers very little to prevent something like this happening here," Richard says.

Instead, it devotes pages to ensuring that doctors and others involved get impunity, Richard says. "The only protection against coercion in this Act is that one doctor [the first doctor who has to assess eligibility] must 'do their best' to detect it in a requesting patient. Frankly, that's a pathetic attempt at protection. There's actually a higher standard of protection available against coercion for the loss of chattels and property in our common law than there is for the loss of human life in the EOLC Act!"

"There's actually a higher standard of protection available against coercion for the loss of chattels and property in our common law than there is for the loss of human life in the EOLC Act!"

Richard says coercion is such a complex issue that our judicial system can spend many weeks in court proceedings grappling with deciding whether it is present in any one property or contract. "Yet David Seymour's Act expects one doctor to achieve in a very short amount of time what our courts spend weeks trying to detect.

"That doctor probably won't even be the person's GP. And how are they supposed to detect coercion? They can't talk to family members of the patient unless the person allows that. And although they can talk to other health practitioners who are in 'regular contact' with the patient, the reality is that many of them [health practitioners] know little or nothing about a patient's family situation, let alone the complex dynamics within their families that might lead to coercion or pressure."

The only accountability and oversight provisions in this Act come in the form of the registrar, who "basically checks if a form has been ticked in the right places", and a "toothless" Review Committee, Richard says.

Richard argues that this law was designed to cater for the Lecretia Seales of this world, for those who are capable, confident and committed. But instead, inadvertently the law will place large numbers of weak, defenceless and vulnerable New Zealanders at risk of being euthanised or helped to die by rogue doctors or abusive family members. "Under this law it will be extremely hard to pin law-breaking on any abusive family members or doctors. There are immunities in the Act that would appear to provide a shield behind which an abuser can easily shelter."

I had personally started to wonder about how doctors engaged in the process would be held accountable, investigated and prosecuted if needed.

Richard says that the concern is a very legitimate one; the only accountability and oversight provisions in this Act come in the form of the registrar, who "basically checks if a form has been ticked in the right places", and a "toothless" Review Committee.

"This Act contains no effective oversight mechanisms for ensuring the accountability of doctors or other people involved in the process. There's no proper way of detecting, preventing or punishing coercion or abuse while it is actually happening."

Many other laws in our country contain much higher levels of monitoring, Richard says. "For example, under the Mental Health Act there are district health inspectors whose job it is to monitor patients being treated or assessed under the Act, checking that correct processes are followed, that patient's rights are respected, and that there's no abuse.

"The closest thing to a monitoring mechanism in the EOLC Act is the registrar whose job primarily is to receive the relevant forms from doctors and check they have been filled in correctly."

As for the Review Committee, it can only inspect cases after the process has been completed. "And we have to ask: what information is that committee given in order to 'review' the cases and process?" The committee is only given a customised report which the doctor has filled in.

"That report won't include any patient records. It'll only contain the patient's name and address, the fact they've died, how the medication was administered, where and when they died and which doctors or nurses were present."

He has an interesting point; even Oregon reports have more information.

"It's what our Review Committee won't be given that concerns me. They won't get any clinical information, or be told the reasons why doctors assessed the patient as eligible, or the reasons why the patient chose euthanasia, or the nature of their 'unbearable suffering'. They won't be told the patient's ethnicity, or socio-economic status, or how effective their healthcare was. And the committee has no powers to make these enquiries of the doctor."

I ask why Richard thinks ethnicity is such an important factor that should be recorded on the forms.

"Currently before the Waitangi Tribunal is a mass claim that the healthcare system is sick and racist, that it's failing Māori in all sectors. Māori are disproportionally represented in our chronic illness, disability,

> **"Elderly, sick Māori are most at risk of being coerced—looking at the elder abuse statistics. They are the ones the health system is failing the most."**

suicide and terminal illness statistics. If there is ever a group to be adversely impacted by the introduction and imposition of this Act it would be Māori. Elderly, sick Māori are most at risk of being coerced—looking at the elder abuse statistics. They are the ones the health system is failing the most. And the same system that is failing them is now going to be the one offering this 'new solution'."

He says it's also important to know these details to see if there are patterns, like a lack of healthcare in certain regions.

So, no one will be monitoring the process in real-time; minimal information will be given to reviewers; coercion detection is sub-par… "What if it's the doctor themselves who's done the coercing? Who would ever know? How would the Review Committee know? There's no way for it to review the doctor's work. There's no possible way to find out from the information they are provided whether the process was done safely for the people who truly wanted it. Their oversight is completely at the mercy of the doctor and whatever information the doctor wants to put into the report. A rogue doctor isn't going to incriminate themselves in their notes."

Why is the process so lacking in transparency? Why are we not provided with information on the reasons behind people making this choice? What suffering was considered unbearable?

"We will have no way of knowing if this law is achieving what it was intended for."

Richard says if someone suspected a doctor of malpractice they would be left with the court system… And courts have made it clear they are extremely cautious about wading into cases involving the health system and based on medical judgements.

"The only other option would be taking a case to the police. But the way the Act works, it will be extremely difficult for police to investigate or prosecute abuses of the process, especially considering that the person has signed forms agreeing to their own death. You'd have to have very compelling evidence—so compelling as to outweigh the quite extensive immunities against liability which doctors are given under the Act."

Is that why there aren't many cases of doctors being prosecuted or found guilty of breaking these laws internationally? "It's certainly one reason."

Richard says a famous end-of-life case was brought before the English House of Lords in the UK in the 1990s, that of Tony Bland v The Airedale NHS Trust. Tony was a crush victim who was left in a vegetative state as a result of injuries he received from metal barriers giving way during a Liverpool football game. He was among a number of others injured in the overcrowded spectator stands. The event was dubbed the 'Hillsborough Disaster'. The hospital, with support from Tony's parents, were applying for permission to end his life.

"The conclusion of the court was that the problem with euthanasia is that when you allow it in any limited set of circumstances, it becomes difficult to see any logical basis for excluding it in others... you've 'crossed the rubicon'. From that point on, there is no going back. What I think New Zealanders have yet to grasp is that the only logical trajectory of a euthanasia law is expansion," Richard says.

"What I think New Zealanders have yet to grasp is that the only logical trajectory of a euthanasia law is expansion."

"That explains why David's claim that no country who's introduced euthanasia has ever gone back. There's only one direction to go in."

The slippery slope argument? "People call it a slippery slope; I call it a logical progression. What we now see happening overseas and find abhorrent, we won't in 10 to 15 years' time if we start down that road ourselves. David calls that 'evolving tikanga' [Māori traditional values]. I call it degradation. We only have to look at the jurisdictions with euthanasia regimes and where they are now three, five or 10 years later and ask ourselves if that is what we want to become."

If the EOLC Act becomes law, Richard predicts that the pro-euthanasia lobby will be the first to push for it to expand, and that within months or a few years we will see another Lecretia Seales-type case involving someone who isn't terminal arguing they should be allowed access to it.

The Crown will know, just like plaintiffs and lawyers, the only reason the EOLC Act had restrictions on eligibility was to cut a political deal to get it passed.

He refers to the Canadian example in which no sooner had the ink dried on their Bill C-14 which allowed medical aid in dying, than there were court challenges by non-terminally-ill Canadians arguing that the new law was discriminatory, Richard says. "And while in New Zealand the law can't be changed without Parliamentary intervention, our courts do have the power to make declarations of inconsistency when they believe something isn't in line with our Bill of Rights Act. The Crown will know, just like plaintiffs and lawyers, the only reason the EOLC Act had restrictions on eligibility was to cut a political deal to get it passed.

"I predict the Crown's going to find itself having to stand before a judge arguing that the law is sufficient, that it isn't too restrictive, and that it shouldn't be expanded. But Crown Law will know, just like the plaintiffs and their lawyers, that the only reason the EOLC Act passed into law with restrictions on eligibility was because David had to cut a political deal in order to get it passed. So, undoubtedly, we'll see declarations of inconsistency in our courts, along with media pressure and societal pressure from its normalisation. This will put a lot of pressure back on Parliament to expand the law."

"Once a euthanasia law passes, the government has to create various apparatus in order to protect and enforce the new 'right' that has been created. So, everybody in every government department, every clinic, hospital, hospice, rest home and retirement village has to fall in line with this new right."

Societal pressure and normalisation have been something observed in the Netherlands, but I question how our society will respond to a law change like this.

"I believe an assisted dying law releases a lot of toxic pathologies into a society, once it gets a hold on it. Once a euthanasia law passes, the government has to create various apparatus in order to protect and enforce the new 'right' that has been created. So, everybody in every government department, every clinic, hospital, hospice, rest home and retirement village has to fall in line with this new right. Laws and policies have to be rewritten. What follows in time is a gradual societal acceptance of the new right. Social mentality changes and the entitlement to euthanasia becomes regarded as a human right.

"That's what we saw in the Canadian courts, where euthanasia quickly became regarded as a 'constitutional right'. It was normalised and became a valid 'healthcare service' which people should be allowed to 'access'... a 'social good'. That's where things start to go awry. You see a gradual promotion of the new 'right' by policymakers. And then you see interest groups and litigants in court arguing why one person should be able to enjoy this 'right' when others are being denied it.

"Over time a social acceptance becomes a social expectation."

So, in law-writing theory—does society have a moral code which is reflected in law, or does law deem morals for society?

"That's a question legal scholars grapple with—the extent to which laws result from social changes and changes in social consciousness, compared to whether they are enacted to effect a change in social consciousness. A lot of laws are the result of a shift of customs, beliefs and so on. Other laws are created by the few and are imposed on the majority in order to change people's perceptions over what is right or wrong."

Richard says the anti-smacking law is a good case in point. "A lot of Kiwis at the time didn't believe smacking was wrong, but then the law changed. And as a result, there was a change in their views—it's now not OK to smack a child. It's a good example that law change is not necessarily a reflection of social beliefs but can be a galvaniser of social change."

> **"At the end of the day the question we are being asked in the upcoming referendum is not if we agree with assisted dying or not, but whether we can live with this law. Quite literally."**

The EOLC Act is just that, Richard says. "David Seymour and a number of parliamentarians, along with at least one sizeable law firm and a 'death with dignity' euthanasia lobby group, have effectively imposed their own version of morality on society through this Act. It's the imposition of David Seymour and Lecretia Seales' views on New Zealand."

So, what does Richard think about the fact that polls show people have been in support of this choice for 20 years? "I don't think the polls are an accurate reflection of what people think the issues are. There are plenty of polls David never mentions to anyone—they are the polls of doctors and palliative care specialists opposed to euthanasia.

"At the end of the day the question we are being asked in the upcoming referendum is not if we agree with assisted dying or not, but whether we can live with this law. Quite literally."

CHAPTER 13:

GRANT ILLINGWORTH QC

Grant Illingworth's home in Epsom is impressively central. It matches my expectations for one of our country's highly-regarded barristers: large, formal... inside gates. Proper, but down-to-earth Grant answers the doorbell and welcomes me into his downstairs office. We sit to discuss a lawmaker's perspective on the Act.

I've read Grant's opinion pieces published by Stuff and have a fair idea that he considers the Act contrary to what good law is intended for. But I want to know why and what exactly it is about this Act that bothers him.

Grant has been practising law in New Zealand for more than 40 years and was appointed as Queen's Counsel in 2003. I ask him to help me better understand his concerns in 'non-legal speech'; really a Legal Guide for Dummies on the EOLC Act.

"It's important to note that Parliament has enacted the End of Life Choice Act on 16 November, 2019. This means that it will automatically come into force if the outcome of the binding referendum is 'yes'. Parliament will not need to review it; it will be introduced in the exact form it's currently in."

Why is that important? "It means that people voting need to fully understand what this exact Act is. It's a finished piece: there is no room for adjustment.

"It's an extraordinary situation really… for an Act to wait for final approval from a binding referendum and immediately become active.

This has never happened in New Zealand before. Normally this decision is made by Parliament."

And to Grant, that isn't a good thing.

"It's a huge concern. The public are being asked to make a legal decision—which is for this particular form of end-of-life choice legislation. How are the public expected to know the legal technicalities? Yet they are actually voting for just that—a set of legal rules that will come into force. The Act contains a number of complicated procedures that the general public can't be expected to understand, certainly not without help."

Grant says these types of Acts are normally considered and dismantled by lawyers and courts as there can be all sorts of subtleties that need to be considered. "In this case it seems the select committee has not really attempted to grapple with the technicalities of the draft that was enacted. In effect, Parliament has passed the buck to the public in relation to an issue that would be called 'quality control for legislation'."

> **"It's a huge concern. The public are being asked to make a legal decision—which is for this particular form of end-of-life choice legislation. How are the public expected to know the legal technicalities?"**

NZ First says the general public are knowledgeable and up with the play; choosing to send it to a referendum is a good act of democracy in their view.

"There's absolutely nothing wrong with referendums being used to determine a policy. But there's a big difference between making a decision on a policy and making a decision on a specific set of rules. If the New Zealand public were being asked, 'Do you think we should have an end-of-life choice? Yes or no' (or something to that effect)—it would be a perfectly good referendum question. But to be asked to sanction an Act of Parliament as a whole is a different thing altogether."

So, from his perspective, is this a good piece of law? I suspect his answer will be no. Grant doesn't mince his words.

"If I thought the process was fine, I wouldn't be here. But it's bad law: it's badly drafted and it's wrong. This is a very serious issue—mistakes about whether to live or die can never be undone. That's why we abolished the death penalty. The legislation must contain safeguards that are so clear and comprehensive that any possibility of deaths occurring by mistake is excluded beyond a reasonable doubt. The EOLC Act fails to meet that standard by a very wide margin."

"If I thought the process was fine, I wouldn't be here. But it's bad law: it's badly drafted and it's wrong. This is a very serious issue—mistakes about whether to live or die can never be undone."

I would expect those words out of an emotional, anti-euthanasia lobbyist's mouth. But here I am sitting with a calm, collected, intelligent and highly-qualified man. He shuffles the papers he is referring to in his hands.

Grant's about to spill into the detail of the errors he sees in the practical application of the Act, step by step. If this referendum gives the go-ahead, this scenario could happen in doctors' clinics around the country.

These are the actual steps laid out in the Act for those wanting assistance in dying:

A person wants to receive assisted dying. They make an appointment with a medical practitioner, most likely their doctor, and inform them of their wish to receive assisted dying (the instigation).

"They don't have to say 'I have a terminal illness'. They don't even have to say 'can you please do an assessment to see if I have an illness'," Grant says.

There is no requirement at this point to assess their eligibility.

Upon receiving the request, the medical practitioner (subject to conscientious objection) has to take the following steps:

1) The medical practitioner must provide some information, first of which is the prognosis for the person's terminal illness…

   So a person can request for assisted dying before they have even been diagnosed with anything? "Under this Act—yes. There's no legal requirement for a person to have an illness before they make that request. They don't even have to ask for an assessment before asking for assisted dying… It's nuts. It starts with an illogical fallacy—someone could ask for something they are not even entitled to. That irrationality progresses throughout the statute."

2) The person must be told about the irreversible nature of dying. "Most people would understand that the nature of dying is irreversible."

3) The doctor must also tell the person of the anticipated impacts of dying… "What exactly is the doctor actually supposed to say? 'It's going to hurt.' Or, 'You're going to be dead.' Or, 'It's going to impact your family'... What are the impacts they are trying to envisage? How is the doctor supposed to know, especially if it's the first time the patient may have met the doctor? And bearing in mind that most doctors in a general practice schedule interviews that run for 10 to 15 minutes."

4) The doctor must communicate with the person at intervals determined by the progress of the person's terminal illness... "Again bearing in mind that they are at this point they are purely assuming the person has a terminal illness."

5) The doctor has to ensure the person understands the other options around their end-of-life care.

6) And ensure the person knows they can change their mind at any time.

7) Encourage that person to discuss their wish with others.

8) Ensure the person knows they are not obliged to discuss it with anyone.

9) The doctor has to do their best to ensure the person expresses their wish free from pressure from any other person.

   The Act says they will do that by conferring with other health practitioners who are in regular contact with the person. They are also to confer with members of the person's family approved by the person.

   "This is the only safeguard to protect people from being pressured to end their lives?... The doctor must 'do their best'?," Grant reels. "If that is a safeguard to protect people from being pressured, that is absolutely and utterly pathetic. It runs against every benefit of the law that protects human life that we have had in our country since the legal system was established. It's hopeless."

"If that is a safeguard to protect people from being pressured, that is absolutely and utterly pathetic."

10) The medical practitioner then gives the person a form to fill in. It is to be signed and dated in front of the doctor then sent to the registrar.

11) After the form has been sent, the practitioner has to then reach the opinion that the person requesting the assisted dying is a person who is eligible...

Yes you read right. After the person has gone through the application process their eligibility is tested.

So, what's wrong here? "Firstly, it's illogical. Secondly, it's a process that has no meaningful safeguards."

Safeguards… a word I've heard tossed around perpetually by David Seymour and those in support who say this Act is tight. But how tight do these safeguards against coercion actually need to be?

"In 45 years of legal practice I have met many, many people who have used pressure, manipulation and all sorts of devious methods to get their own way. There are many, many people in our community willing to do that to get a person's money. It's utterly naive to think this statute contains sufficient safeguards to protect people from that pressure. You only have to think for a moment what the financial benefits can be if a vulnerable person has life insurance, or owns property, to realise this is a real problem.

"The opportunity is there, the ability to hide it is there—the only question is: are there really people out there who will do this? And the answer is—that's why the criminal courts are full every day of people being sentenced for wrongdoing. There are heaps of people in our community willing to do wrong things to achieve advantage for themselves."

Of note, doctors can opt out of this whole procedure at the initial stages by using conscientious objection, which basically means they pass the case on to the approved agency who will redistribute the patient to someone else. But there are some questions around what is classed as conscientious objection and if that would be broad enough to cover someone who just doesn't want to be involved in assisting someone to die.

"There are various kinds of conscientious objection rights recognised in different statutes. But even there are still limits. Does it have to be religious or ethical beliefs for it to be valid?"

Grant says the whole process puts doctors in a difficult position. "Is it really right for a doctor to proceed through the assisted dying process on the basis that a person has a terminal illness when that assumption may be incorrect? Does the doctor have to provide a diagnosis of an illness they have no experience about?"

The process could be abused by doctors, but what the legislation itself requires is an abuse of doctors, he says. "This law would contradict and override medical standards and ethics. If it hasn't been approved by medical tribunals, how are they going to deal with it when there are disputes and complaints made against their doctors? If the law conflicts with the standards of the medical profession, then the law is stupid."

Grant puts down the papers he's been working through. His eyes flicker as he reflects.

"I find it hard to believe this is the law we are voting on... the only thing that will stand in the way of someone's death. It's just so poorly thought through about the logic of the process."

"I find it hard to believe this is the law we are voting on... the only thing that will stand in the way of someone's death. It's just so poorly thought through about the logic of the process. Surely if the steps are illogical and you're talking about an issue of life and death it should raise the question: has this been thought through properly? Has whoever drafted this legislation actually put their brain into gear?"

If this law truly is defective, I wonder why it hasn't been picked up and analysed by the Justice Select Committee. Why wasn't it scrutinised, or at least why weren't changes made through the third reading process by MPs? Why didn't the lawyers who have surely looked over this legislation raised any of these issues?

"I'm looking at it with 45 years of legal training. I can possibly see things others possibly don't see. That's not being immodest: it's

"The question is: could this law be abused and result in people dying who shouldn't? The answer is simply, 'yes'. It's an incredibly dangerous piece of legislation."

simply saying legal training does have some benefit when trying to interpret legislation. I'm sure they have engaged lawyers in this but I just don't think the legal advice or drafting has been good enough to produce a quality outcome—which is essential in a case where life-and-death issues are being addressed.

"My concern in this case is not so much about the rights and wrongs of assisted dying. I have my personal views, but what I'm pointing to is the fact that if you're going to have a law of this kind it should involve a rational process and the drafting of the statute needs to be done with particular care. I believe this legislation doesn't reach that standard. I believe it falls so far below that standard it is simply not fit for purpose."

I don't understand how Lecretia Seales and her law friends who so adamantly supported this law thought it was good practice.

"Well it's a hugely emotional issue. And people's clarity of thinking can become clouded simply because it's a battle they want to succeed in. They're interested in the principle and not the detail. But the details are important because it's a matter of life and death. People will die as a result of this badly-drafted statute," he says. "Most of the people who will die, if this gets voted through, will be within the spirit of what was intended. But the question is: could this law be abused and result in people dying who shouldn't? The answer is simply, 'yes'. It's an incredibly dangerous piece of legislation."

The weightiness of his statement lingers. For the first time I feel the depth of this referendum decision, as though this could truly be a turning point in history. I'm not sure if it is because I trust Grant's assessment, or whether I've been sucked into his convincing argument... or if I'm actually realising the magnitude and potential this law change could have on people. I try not to let it disturb my thoughts as I direct the interview in a slightly different direction.

Several times through the journey of discovery so far I've wondered how the concept of freedom of choice interacts with law. How do we have freedom to decide what we want when there's obviously the law of the land at work? How do we make law that doesn't impede on people's rights? And in a day where 'my body, my choice' is becoming the mantra of the moment, how does law allow for this when it decides what is and isn't allowed for everyone?

Grant gently takes me through a basic understanding of the motivation of law.

"If we go back to the 1600s, which is a long way back, there was a very important case called Calvin's Case. It was in England. The courts in England essentially said that people who are subject to the laws of the country owe a duty of allegiance to the Crown. Essentially this means you have a duty to be loyal to the Queen and representatives. And on the other side of the coin is that the Crown has a duty of protection. That duty of protection has been part of the obligation of the governments for centuries. It's recognised in section eight of the Bill of Rights Act of New Zealand. So, every citizen, every permanent resident, and indeed every visitor, has the right to be protected by the Crown and its agencies.

"If Parliament is authorising doctors to kill people without appropriate safeguards, then the Crown has breached the obligation which has existed for hundreds of years."

"That's why we have a police force. When someone takes a gun and tries to murder people in a mosque the police turn out in force and protect our community. They are fulfilling the Crown's obligation to protect us."

So protection is a foundational principle in good lawmaking?

"That's why to suggest people can be killed without adequate safeguards means we have forgotten that fundamental aspect of our community arrangements. We've forgotten that the Crown has a duty to safeguard life and make sure those safeguards are effective and appropriate. If Parliament is authorising doctors to kill people without appropriate safeguards, then the Crown has breached the obligation which has existed for hundreds of years.

"Basically it all comes down to one thing... does this statute safeguard human life in the way it should? And the answer to that is a big fat 'no'."

Autonomy and law are a funny combination. Trying to combine them is like mixing water and oil.

Most of us Kiwis like to live 'each to their own', except if there's a breach in level-four lockdown protocol (when we'd happily report a law-breaking citizen).

We are fiercely independent. And righteously indignant against judgmentalism. We don't like it if someone tells us what to do. And we don't like telling others what to do. It's 'live and let live', where tolerance is king.

That's the water. So, what's the oil? Batting for the underdog, and sticking up for the little guy. Protecting the weak and defending the marginalised. Ensuring everybody has been heard and all play a part. Social equality. That's true democracy after all.

Lawmaking seems to have to constantly balance these two weights... law and personal freedom. In fact, now I think of it, that's what the universal symbol for law is—the scales of justice.

Because we are engaging in a referendum of a legal nature we have been granted permission to consider whether this Act is good for someone else. Not only do we have permission, but we should be compelled to also assess its impacts on others.

Am I my brother's keeper? Yes. In lawmaking you are.

Do we have responsibility to decide what is good and evil? Yes. In lawmaking you do.

How am I going to do that? Learn. And vote.

CHAPTER 14: ROBERT PRESTON

The United Kingdom has constantly rejected its equivalent version of assisted dying laws when they have reached Parliament, the most recent in 2015. It is one of more than 30 nations and jurisdictions to dismiss attempts to introduce law changes in favour. A man who knows all the ins and outs of the UK's stance, Robert Preston, is fielding my Skype call.

Robert was a senior civil servant in Whitehall for 33 years and a committee clerk in the House of Lords. As part of his role, he accompanied a committee reviewing assisted dying laws operating in the United States, the Netherlands and Switzerland. The committee also interviewed more than 150 expert witnesses and read over 12,000 letters from members of the public in Britain on the issue before writing a report summarising its findings. The report was presented to Parliament, which in turn rejected subsequent bills on assisted dying.

Robert retired, but two years later he was shoulder-tapped to help start a think tank called Living and Dying Well. He insisted that his involvement depended on the organisation not being a campaigning group.

"I believe there are respectable arguments on both sides of this debate and I was tired of all the mudslinging between them."

His thoughts on our impending vote?

"My view is the status quo should not be changed. It is just fine as it is; it's just right. There are serious dangers in changing the law."

He says this is true for both his home nation and ours.

"In saying that, the evidence is not all one way. I try to be objective and respect the other side's point of view; unfortunately some campaigning groups don't."

I can't help but relate to what Robert is saying. He states there are three tests that would have to be passed before assisted dying could be responsibly licensed by law. He suggests we start with the law, as this is the key to understanding the debate.

"What is being proposed is a change in the law—so, what is the law? Very few people understand that. The law in New Zealand is very similar to the law in Britain—encouraging or assisting suicide is illegal.

"The purpose of the law is to outlaw practices which are harmful to society. There are penalties for people who do that out of criminal intent. But there is also discretion for prosecutors where it is very clear there is no criminal intent and the circumstances are exceptional. That's the way we deal with any law."

Robert says nobody would want to see a mother who has no money and steals because she is desperate to feed her child prosecuted in a heavy-handed way. Nor would anyone want to see a father speeding in his car rushing to take his child to hospital prosecuted harshly. "We look to see exceptional cases dealt with exceptionally, and that's what the law does right now. That's totally different to what is being proposed.

"What's being proposed is creating a licensing system whereby, provided you are thought to have fulfilled a certain number of criteria, you can go ahead and do this with impunity. We do not license by law acts that are generally harmful to society, but which, in highly exceptional circumstances, may be forgivable."

There are three tests that have to be passed before a law should be changed, Robert says. "The first is you need to show that the current law is not working."

And you would say ours is? "Yes."

Those in favour of assisted dying would beg to differ. Let's say the current law fails the first test; I'm curious to hear what Robert's second test is.

"Can you do it safely?"

The question of safeguards...

"I've looked at the legislation in New Zealand and they are not safeguards at all. They are a checklist; a tick-box list that a doctor will have to say 'yes' to. For example, is this person being pressured? How would they know that? My doctor has said to me quite frankly, 'I wouldn't have a clue if you were being pressured'. Many doctors only really know what the patient tells them when it comes to social or personal questions like this."

Robert says it may be possible to tighten up some of the safeguards by taking the process out of the hands of doctors and giving it to a senior court. "The court would then take evidence from the medical profession, psychiatrists, meet the family and make an all-round decision after an exhaustive process."

Wouldn't that process be too long for someone with only six months to live? "The courts can actually accelerate things. The point is, if you give the decision to the court, it makes someone considering ending their life think very carefully before going ahead. It's important not to make the process too easy."

The way it stands, the doctor is the judge, jury and executioner. And also the witness.

The way it stands, the doctor is the judge, jury and executioner. And also the witness. Something that most doctors in Britain would refuse to sign up for, and in Oregon, many avoid.

"A recent survey of GPs carried out in Britain showed only 14 per cent of those questioned would be prepared to conduct an examination of all the social and medical factors and decide on 'assisted dying',"

Robert says. "That means people would have to hunt around to find a doctor who will do it. It's been coined 'doctor shopping'."

Doesn't that have an impact on getting an objective assessment? "Exactly. This isn't a job for the medical profession. If you have a court-based system the doctor would simply give advice on strictly medical issues. Is this person terminally ill? How much longer do they have to live? What other care can be given?"

"A couple of years ago a Swedish researcher got in touch with the Oregon Health Department and asked whether an insulin-dependent diabetes patient would qualify for assisted dying if he stopped taking his insulin and became terminal. They said, 'Yes'. So if you hadn't been diagnosed as terminal but could make yourself... that would count."

Robert says that's the third test—explain why this is a job for the medical profession.

"It isn't a medical issue but a social issue for discussion by a court not the medical profession. It's the role of the courts to balance rights for some against protection for others."

It's an interesting concept moving the application process from the medical field to the courtroom. But no other nation that has introduced the law has made that move. I wonder whether there's a standout point he has observed from all the nations he has visited and studied on this issue.

"There is one thing that keeps coming up... the change in law. There is constant pressure to extend existing assisted dying laws. Within the last 10 years in Oregon there have been three or four attempts. And the interpretation of how the law is applied is what you also have to watch."

I ask for an example and Oregon again is offered. Oregon's assisted suicide criteria include a prognosis of terminal illness within six months. "A couple of years ago a Swedish researcher got in touch with the Oregon Health Department and asked whether an insulin-dependent diabetes patient would qualify for assisted dying if he stopped taking his insulin and became terminal. They said, 'Yes'. So if you hadn't been diagnosed as terminal but could make yourself… that would count."

Robert says the law as it stands in our countries has a rational boundary. "As one parliamentarian so well put: laws are like nation states—they are more secure when their boundaries rest on natural frontiers. The law we have now rests on such a frontier. It rests on the principle that we do not involve ourselves in deliberately bringing about the deaths of other people. Once you abandon that principle and introduce arbitrary criteria like terminal illness, that boundary becomes just a line in the sand, easily crossed and hard to defend.

"At the moment you can defend the law's criteria because they are natural criteria. But the minute you start changing that, you open a can of worms. There's no rational boundary; that is why these laws tend to get extended."

Robert says he has been shocked at how everyone struggles to keep an objective view on the issue. "You can't make law based on just your own story. People have asked me if I would want this [assisted dying] for myself. I honestly don't know... but the fact that I might want it for myself is not a reason to change the law."

The reason why people want it is not often exposed. "Those in favour say they want it for people who die in agony. In the 1950s, people often did die in pain as we didn't have the expertise to relieve it. Now, science has advanced in leaps and bounds. And yet now we are talking about assisted dying. This is a paradox. Science has gone the opposite way than the campaigning. It's a curiosity really."

Long-lasting illnesses are also more common and death has slowed, causing more mental distress like frustration, Robert says. "It's a change in the pattern of dying."

He has a good understanding of the historical context we are in regarding assisted dying. I'm not going to say it's because he's 75, but honestly it does help. Robert's comments reverberated with Margo Somerville's opinion..."We need to ask 'why now?'".

"When I was a boy people died regularly and we were accustomed to death. My parents had to fight through two world wars, and through the Depression. There was no free medical healthcare. They just accepted death as part of life. People used to die pretty young. My grandfather died at 67 and people said that was a good innings. Now we put death out of our minds because we don't see it enough. When it does happen we put it in the hands of hospitals, carers, doctors and funeral directors.

"People have asked me if I would want this [assisted dying] for myself. I honestly don't know... but the fact that I might want it for myself is not a reason to change the law."

"It's something to be forgotten about when you are healthy, and resented when your health fails. We've become accustomed to controlling our lives in all sorts of ways. But with dying, we've come up against something we can't control. And we don't like it.

"I remember one doctor wrote that nowadays death seems to be resented by people. When he told people they were terminally ill, it's not so much they were sad but that it was unfair. They've grown up thinking life should be wonderful. If that's your mindset, then when you die it will seem unfair."

Control and autonomy often go hand in hand throughout the discussion on assisted dying. And it seems to be a recurring philosophy that is being widely used across a number of issues in society. Why?

"As we grow more prosperous we feel we are in control, and when we come across something we can't control we become frustrated."

"To some extent it comes from rising levels of prosperity. I'm certainly not against prosperity, but as we grow more prosperous we feel we are in control, and when we come across something we can't control we become frustrated.

"A good example is my life in many ways: I'm a member of what's been called the 'lucky generation'. I was born at the end of the war, I had a free university education with no fees, there was guaranteed entry into the professions, a good salary. It's this generation that is at the forefront for these demands. We've got used to having it all our own way.

"Prosperity makes us not want to be dependent on others. And we don't want others to be dependent on us. Illness is one of those things that shatters that illusion."

CHAPTER 15:

PAULA TESORIERO MNZM

"Personal Account

The illusion of self-reliance has already been shattered for those within the disability community. It's something they have had to let go of when confronted with restrictions surrounding their life circumstances. The reality is, at times this has left them feeling extremely vulnerable.

Vulnerable isn't a very popular label to own. It carries a fair amount of negative publicity and usually has an association with weakness. Its interpretation is as vast as the word 'suffering'. David Seymour doesn't like the adjective much. In relation to assisted dying, he says it's a term volleyed around like a ping-pong ball.

But when motivational factors that propel people into considering assisted dying include loss of autonomy and 'dignity', the feeling of being a burden, suffering, pain… it's clear this is something that will impact the disabled community directly. These are issues they face every day.

Disabled people often also experience depression, grief, shock and loss. Many are considered 'terminal', or can become terminal at any time, either by the progression of their illness or by their own choice to refuse treatment, medication or care. They already grapple with a sense of disqualification and misunderstanding and feel the weight of judgment around measuring 'quality of life' by the ability to function. They face accessibility restrictions, in a physical sense, but also from a lack of funding to gain equipment and care they need to live life to the fullest.

They are qualified to say something about the EOLC Act. That view is certainly supported by New Zealand Disability Rights Commissioner Paula Tesoriero.

Right out of the gate Paula Tesoriero wants to make it clear that people need to know we will be voting on a specific piece of legislation in the upcoming referendum, not on whether we agree with assisted dying. "We need to get our heads around the Act, not the philosophical issue." A law graduate from Victoria University, Paula has worked in private practice and as a General Manager at Statistics NZ and the Ministry of Justice.

In her role as Disability Rights Commissioner, Paula advocates for the rights of New Zealand's population who are disabled. One in four New Zealanders has a disability. Impairments may be physical, sensory, neurological, psychiatric or intellectual. The vast majority of those disabled people who have contacted her about this issue are not in favour of this Act.

Paula not only brings a commentary on behalf of the disability sector to the table, but also her own personal experience. She's a gold-winning and world-record-breaking Paralympics cyclist. And an amputee.

Paula had three of her limbs affected by Amniotic Band Syndrome, a rare condition caused when a developing foetus gets exposed to fibrous amniotic bands which wrap themselves around the baby's body. "It restricts the blood flow, which results in amputation or not enough blood supply to form in the way most babies form," Paula says. "In relation to me it affected my right hand… my thumb is really the only finger that looks like most other people's hands. Both my legs were affected. My left leg had a foot, but I couldn't walk on it. When

I was 13 a decision was made to amputate that below the knee. My right leg has no functioning ankle; the circulation below the knee is not very good."

This meant as a child Paula couldn't keep up with other kids' running and walking. She was acutely aware she was different, but she discovered her bike gave her a sense of freedom and "fitting in". "I used to ride [my bike] everywhere, daring to imagine that I might become one of the fastest people in the world on a bike."

That dream drove her to confront her own disability. And while her dreams came true at the Beijing Summer Paralympics in 2008 when she won the women's 500m time trial, her proudest achievement was facing her own fears.

"When I stood in a Paralympic village for the first time, I finally understood I am not who I am despite my disability—I am who I am because of my disability."

> **"When I stood in a Paralmypic village for the first time, I finally understood I am not who I am despite my disability—I am who I am because of my disability."**

Paula's services to cycling were recognised when she was made a Member of the New Zealand Order of Merit in 2009, retiring as an athlete in 2010.

So when a law is being discussed that directly interacts with discourses surrounding disability, it's no wonder the topic is tender. Paula says many have found even the pretext of discussions around assisted dying personally insulting.

Why is it particularly troubling? "Because of the association of dignity with independence and because disabled people may be one of the most at-risk groups for coercion."

And that is something that most people fail to understand or recognise or acknowledge, Paula says. When the top motivational

> **"It was insulting to hear the comments made by MPs in the chamber reflecting on seeing the reality of loved ones losing independence and dignity because someone had to care for them."**

factors in people choosing assisted dying in overseas jurisdictions include loss of independence, being unable to participate in community, loss of control and becoming a burden on others, then the disabled community rightfully has a reason to be concerned.

"This is something many disabled people deal with every day," Paula says. "Much of what we heard in Parliament during debates on the EOLC Bill was talk around the issues of dignity being associated with loss of control which happens around the end of someone's life… This loss of control can be a daily existence for disabled people.

"What message does it send when an MP describes a family member's loss of control as undignified? What message does it send when we introduce a law like this where internationally people choose to use assisted suicide and euthanasia because of this perceived indignity?"

Paula says it was insulting to hear the comments made by MPs in the chamber reflecting on seeing the reality of loved ones losing independence and dignity because someone had to care for them.

"Judging by my own social media posts those comments were hurtful and they had an effect on the disabled community. Many have been offended about what has been said in these debates and the apparent dismissal of concerns of the disabled community.

"You have to consider what message it sends to legalise something like this."

Granted, the eligibility criteria does not allow someone to qualify for assisted dying purely because of a disability... but for many impairments there is no bright-line test distinguishing them from a terminal condition, Paula says. "There are many types of impairments that by their very nature are terminal. The point at which someone becomes certain they are within the six-month prognosis is not clear. There's no bright-line test between them. It's kind of like the 'togs, togs, undies' ad that used to be on TV…"

These factors mean a number of disabled people are very likely to be eligible, or become eligible very easily. And they are also the most likely to feel vulnerable to coercion. "We can't pretend some won't be disproportionately impacted by this law. There are people with certain impairments who can be more vulnerable around coercion, like older people with dementia or people with learning disabilities."

The safeguards in law that involve life and death must be watertight and they aren't, Paula says. "Coercion already exists in daily life for some with disabilities. Some of that comes from families; there can also be a lack of understanding within the medical profession of what it is like to live as a disabled person. All of those factors get played out when it comes to an end-of-life regime."

"There are many types of impairments that by their very nature are terminal. The point at which someone becomes certain they are within the six-month prognosis is not clear. There's no bright-line test between them. It's kind of like the 'togs, togs, undies' ad that used to be on TV…"

Paula says one doctor's attempt to 'do their best' is not satisfactory enough to find pressure on a person, especially if the doctor does not have a good understanding of an impairment. "The process is minimal at best. Limiting enquiries to just those

"At no point is the person assessed for their mental health condition or physical health condition that may affect judgment, behaviour or decision-making."

'approved by the person' [applying for assisted dying] will rule out a whole group of people who are often the ones involved in raising concerns about coercion—like neighbours, social workers, district nurses, care providers and extended family. It's possible you'll be left with the group that are most likely the protagonists in the situation."

Paula has major concerns around the assessment of competency in the Act as it is more likely to impact on disabled people. "We do have to respect people who are competent to make decisions but that isn't always clear. There's no adequate check and balance."

According to the Act, a person is considered competent if they have an ability to understand the nature of assisted dying and its consequences. "This is an extremely simplistic definition which falls well short of common interpretations of what competency is, both in a legal and clinical sense. At no point is the person assessed for their mental health condition or physical health condition that may affect judgment, behaviour or decision-making. Even if the patient gets referred to a specialist for further testing—like the Act says a doctor could do—there is no required assessment of these factors. An individual could experience severe depression or be affected by potentially transient factors such as fear, despair or loneliness yet still be able to pass the Act's 'competence' test."

There's also a number of safeguards missing. "There's no judicial oversight. There's no disabled person representation included in the SCENZ Group, there's no 'cooling off' period for those applying for assisted dying. Internationally a number of laws include a period of days or weeks before applications for assisted dying can be fulfilled to prevent emotional decision-making.

"The cooling-off period is especially important with disabled people. There are countless situations where someone goes through tough times of real challenges with impairment. If their impairment is caused by an accident, it's often in the early days. But people do emerge from it… You don't want people at a vulnerable time to make a fatal decision."

Overly simplistic wording, poor definitions and weak processes are a result of a haphazard formation of the law due to the political process it went through during its formation, Paula says. "Our system let us down this time. The Select Committee essentially put the law-writing back onto Parliament after a few tweaks and commentary. And as a result there was a huge amount of SOPs put through. The SOPs that were passed had impacts and implications on other parts of the Bill, affecting the sense of cohesion.

"In Victoria, Australia, when they started developing their legislation they co-designed it. They had disabled people, palliative care, ethicists, lawyers all inputting from the beginning. Their legislation is four times longer than ours. The level of complexity and detail their legislation goes into shows that ours is seriously lacking."

"The cooling-off period is especially important with disabled people. There are countless situations where someone goes through tough times of real challenges with impairment. If their impairment is caused by an accident, it's often in the early days. But people do emerge from it…"

While the legislation itself is inadequate the debate around freedom of choice is ill-informed. Paula says people also need to recognise we aren't all on the same level playing field when it comes to someone's 'right to choose'.

"Choice in the context of disability is an interesting concept. It's misleading to say we are all on a level playing field... Many disabled people don't get to make choices on a daily basis about who they live with, where they live, whether they consent to medical treatment, or about service provision. This debate is taking place in the absence of discussion on access and adequacy of care.

"We really do live in a country that has some quite ableist views and a very medicalised model of disabilities… one that tries to fix the disability rather than a social model that looks at how we break down the barriers around us so disabled people can live the best lives possible. This underlying premise is found everywhere."

Paula fires me a list of stats that demonstrate the differences already present between disabled and non-disabled people… Disabled people face twice the unemployment rate than the usual numbers, 36 per cent of young disabled people are not engaged in education, training, or employment; health outcomes, particularly for those with learning disabilities, fare worse.

Disabled people are over-represented in the youth justice system. Disabled women are twice as likely to be subject to violence and abuse. Accessible housing in New Zealand is a real concern with two per cent of housing stock accessible, and cities and infrastructure are not as accessible as they should be. Simply getting out and about for many can be challenging. "These demonstrate systemic and structural ableism."

Paula says one piece of international evidence which should be held in high regard comes from the United Nations Human Rights Special Rapporteur report released in April 2019. The UN independent expert Catalina Devandas Aguilar advises on progress, opportunities and challenges encountered in the implementation of the rights of disabled people worldwide. After several weeks in Canada she released a report as a summary of her findings.

The report stated:

"I am extremely concerned about the implementation of the legislation on medical assistance in dying from a disability perspective. I have been informed that there is no protocol in place to demonstrate that persons with disabilities have been provided with viable alternatives when eligible for assistive dying. I have further received worrisome claims about persons with disabilities in institutions being pressured to seek medical assistance in dying, and practitioners not formally reporting cases involving persons with disabilities. I urge the Federal Government to investigate these complaints and put into place adequate safeguards to ensure that persons with disabilities do not request assistive dying simply because of the absence of community-based alternatives and palliative care."

"I have further received worrisome claims about persons with disabilities in institutions being pressured to seek medical assistance in dying, and practitioners not formally reporting cases involving persons with disabilities," says UN expert Catalina Devandas Aguilar.

Paula says it is premature to have an assisted dying regime ahead of resolving issues around adequate support for disabled people to live good lives.

I ask Paula if she thinks there will be pressure from the pro-assisted dying lobby group for eligibility criteria to change if the EOLC Act passes, possibly to re-include the grievous and irremediable illness clause.

"I think we could see an argument for its extension. There are many examples of laws changing as society changes. People start to get used to the idea and then it's easier to relax its stance around it and open things up. David Seymour received criticism for narrowing the scope from those in favour of the law change."

Before we end, I ask Paula to give me her definition of dignity—both for me as a non-disabled person to get a better understanding from a different perspective, and to address those who are within the 'disability' community to offer a better foundation.

"Dignity is being able to live the kind of life you want to live. For many people, that may require additional support. And that's OK. But dignity is about making sure people have what they need in order to live a good life. Just because you're disabled doesn't mean you can't live a good life.

"Disabled people do live great lives."

I am increasingly aware of my ignorance when it comes to those suffering every day with disabilities.

I think most of us Kiwis would say one of the trademarks we're proud of is our independence. Maybe it's because we are a little island off in the corner of the world, doing our own thing. It's forced us to foster skills with the ol' 'number 8 wire'... we've had to make things work ourselves. I think somehow it's become part of the fabric of our mindset that it's best not to need anyone. Having a baby hit that sentiment head-on for me.

One of the most beautiful parts of having a newborn is the awe that this precious life is completely trusting and reliant on you as a parent. It's strange to think this is beautiful in one context, but supposedly ugly in another. It makes me wonder if dignity really is tied to independence? Is value and quality of life also bound to it?

In our fast-paced world of getting things done, productivity being success, and more is best; having someone reliant on you is like having a crutch. It's an attitude I have to confront in myself. And I think it's one that could easily create pressure when someone's considering the timing of death.

SECTION 5:

INTERNATIONAL COMPARISONS

It's a minefield. It's essential we consider the application of assisted dying laws internationally, but it's a complex task when the variables are so vast.

Not only are the laws written slightly differently in each nation, but also the records and reporting processes are all over the show, and trying to measure things such as a shift in cultural perception is convoluted.

Like in every other part of this discussion, those in favour of the law present a very tidy, simplistic statement.

Claims are made that: "No other law has been changed or revoked in any other jurisdiction. No medical practitioner anywhere has been charged with misconduct. The law is doing what it was intended to do."

But further inspection shows it just isn't that clear-cut. For a start, I quickly found the number of the nations who have rejected assisted dying laws far outnumber those that have accepted them.

The amount of analysis and reviews on the laws could fill a library. So my focus is to gain a basic understanding of the most closely associated laws and nations to ours. To see who has been using it, and why. Whether processes are being followed and abuses being caught. To consider the impact on the medical field, and find out whether or not safeguards are working.

The physically closest jurisdiction to home which has introduced an assisted dying law is the state of Victoria in Australia. It's also one of the most recent to legalise it. There it's regarded as one of the most rigorous and comprehensive laws. It allows for assisted suicide, not euthanasia. It has 68 safeguards and the law-writing process included input from an array of affected groups including doctors, disability representatives and ethicists.

As it has only been in operation since June 2019 it is hard to pull much information from the region, but one figure that was surprising was around the level of uptake. The Victorian Government predicted 12 people would use it in the first year, one a month, as people got used to the idea. But 52 had used it in the first six months.

Some would say that this is a good thing. Maybe the result of it being so widely publicised and understood... that it is needed. As with many things, it depends on how you look at it.

Case in point is Dr Stephanie Green and Dr Leonie Herx. They are prominent doctors who have visited New Zealand to engage in our debate. Both have very direct involvement with the practice in their home country of Canada. Stephanie has provided euthanasia for over 150 people. Leonie is a professor of palliative care at Queen's University. Yet they sit on opposite ends.

"There is no evidence of expansion, of eligibility criteria anywhere, being considered. There's no evidence of any misuse or abuse of the system. We have over 8,000 deaths and no clinician or healthcare professional has been charged with abuse or misuse of the system," says Stephanie.

"Two-and-a-half years after its legalisation in Canada, strong lobbies are intensifying their push for euthanasia as a response to mental illness, physical disability, cognitively incapacitated patients through advance directives, and children. Other jurisdictions need to take a hard look at the reality of the Canadian context before holding Canada up as an example to be emulated," says Leonie.

Help?!... I'm going to need some assistance untangling the tentacles of these two doctors.

What is happening overseas? And what can we learn?

CHAPTER 16:

JANE SILLOWAY-SMITH

It's probably a good move to get an American to wade in between two opposing Canadians and act as a mediator. So I've called on California-based researcher Jane Silloway-Smith to help me understand why doctors Stephanie Green and Leonie Herx dispute facts on the same law and system used within their own country.

"Two people can look at the exactly the same set of facts and come to two very different conclusions about what the facts are telling us. They can only begin to tell a story once you give them context," Jane says.

Jane knows the context. She is bringing nearly a decade of study on assisted dying to the table. A public policy researcher who specialises in issues of social justice, Jane began her career here in New Zealand at Maxim Institute. After seven years she branched off on her own and established Every Life Research Institute, dedicating her energy entirely to bioethical policy issues, especially euthanasia. In 2018 she moved back to the United States with her husband and three kids where she continues her work.

Jane's thorough research and understanding on international jurisdictions is invaluable. We're talking via Skype and we are entering a domain Jane is enthusiastic about. We've got a couple of hours while her two-year-old naps.

Let's start with Canada. This is the country whose law ours is based on.

David Seymour has strong ties with Canada having spent time there in his early career working for think tank Frontier Centre for Public

Policy. In fact, there's a video circulating of David in his younger years doing a Canadian News interview in a Canadian accent; it provides a chuckle.

I can understand why he puts the 'eh' into his accent—my two brothers moved to the United States 11 years ago and were so frustrated by not being understood they rolled their R's just to avoid being asked to repeat themselves. Of course when I chatted with them on the phone I wanted to smack the American out of them.

New Zealanders can relate to Canada. We are a lot like them; we are both progressive, have beautiful backyards… and also have 'interesting' neighbours (America and Australia, respectively).

Assisted dying laws in Canada gained momentum in 2015 after their Supreme Court in the Carter v Canada case ruled that prohibition on assisted suicide was overly broad and it unduly abridged people's rights.

The case was made by two women suffering from degenerative diseases who wanted access to assisted suicide, that the law that prohibited euthanasia was unconstitutional. "It was a similar case as that of Lecretia Seales'," Jane says.

The court struck down the prohibition and gave the Canadian Parliament a year to draft a new law to govern an assisted dying regime.

In 2016 the Canadian Parliament legalised what they call "medical assistance in dying" or MAID. To access it a person must be at least 18 years old, have a serious and incurable disease or disability, be in an advanced state of irreversible decline, be enduring physical and psychological suffering which is intolerable, and have their natural death be "reasonably foreseeable".

The law was rushed in because of the deadline, Jane says. To add to the chaos, they had elections and a change in government part of the way through the law forming process. "While Parliament had the power to pass the new law, it was left to the several provinces and their health bodies, medical colleges, and hospital networks to figure out exactly how it was going to work."

There were many Canadian news articles from that time detailing how disruptive and complicated the process was for the medical profession, Jane says. "There was a scramble. Hospitals, hospices and doctors had to decide if they were going to do it, and how. From an administrator's perspective it was a nightmare. It's like being told that how you do medicine is going to change… tomorrow. It was extremely complicated."

She says doctors could opt-in to take part, and many did at first. "But after performing one euthanasia a significant number of doctors asked to have their names removed from the lists. A lot of doctors said they found it extraordinarily distressing."

"But after performing one euthanasia a significant number of doctors asked to have their names removed from the lists. A lot of doctors said they found it extraordinarily distressing."

That's not surprising to Jane, who says the practice of euthanasia isn't that different from being involved in applying the death penalty via lethal injection. "It's the same process—you put a wrap around their arm, you place them in a coma, and then you give them lethal drugs to stop their heart and their breathing. The drugs are often the same, too. In applying the death penalty, however, the state doesn't put the onus of ending another person's life on just one doctor the way it does with euthanasia. The psychology of ending another person's life is fraught.

"Firing squads have several people with guns, only one of which is loaded with real bullets—so no one knows who really killed the person. They do this to provide emotional relief to the executioners."

I wondered whether Jane was adding a touch of American drama to her research. So I looked into it.

In 2017, Canadian newspaper *The National Post* reported that a number of doctors in Canada who had helped end lives were no longer willing to participate in assisted death because of emotional distress or fear of prosecution.

In Ontario, one of the few provinces to track the information, 24 doctors were permanently removed from a voluntary referral list of physicians willing to help people die. Another 30 have put their names on temporary hold, according to a health ministry spokesman. That left 137 doctors on the list willing to provide it. And 30 of those doctors would only provide a second patient assessment, not administer the injection.

Other interesting results appeared. After the first nine months from when the law was introduced, in the Quebec region there were 262 euthanasia deaths—three times more than predicted. And of those, 21 cases were found to be non-compliant. Most of those cases breached the requirement of two doctors assessing the patient, as the doctors were considered not sufficiently independent. Two other patients who had been given euthanasia were not at the 'end-of-life', while a third didn't have a serious or incurable condition. None of the doctors involved faced the discipline committee.

So some drama seemed to be legitimate.

Moving on to neighbour nation America, more than nine States have adopted laws allowing for assisted suicide, not euthanasia. These include: Oregon, Washington, Washington DC, California, Colorado, Hawaii, Maine, New Jersey and Vermont. Interestingly more than 26 States have rejected it.

Requirements include that patients must be 18 or over, competent, and terminally ill with a prognosis of six months or less. They must request the prescription from a doctor multiple times, both in writing and orally, with a cooling-off period of 15 days between requests. They must have a second opinion and may require a psychiatrist's report. The drugs must be self-administered. Doctors who object offering assisted suicide don't have to refer their patients to someone who will do it.

Once you've received the prescription drugs from the pharmacy, there are no conditions on how, when or where you can take them, other than it can't be done in a public place. Recording details surrounding the death is not mandatory.

Jane says, "This means there are people living with lethal drugs just sitting in their medicine cabinet. No one has to be there when the person takes them or dies. It really is a terrifying regime they have. Because often no one is present, you don't know whether the patient ingested the drugs themselves, or by accident, or if they suffered complications. Or whether someone else was involved in administering the drugs."

I ask Jane what she means by 'complications'.

"States like Oregon that have recorded around six per cent of patients have suffered complications after taking the drugs. Within that six per cent there are people who have gone into a coma for two days and then regained consciousness. The most common complication is people regurgitating them... You have to remember these are really lethal drugs your body doesn't want inside of itself."

"Within that six per cent there are people who have gone into a coma for two days and then regained consciousness. The most common complication is people regurgitating them... You have to remember these are really lethal drugs your body doesn't want inside of itself."

Gross.

Oregon and Washington have the best statistics available from the legalised States as they've had it operating for the longest time. Oregon passed the law in '97 and

The reasons for people choosing to use it is also very different to the original assumption that pain would be a motivational factor.

it was operational from '98.

Since it was first introduced, there has only been one amendment to the law in Oregon—and that was to the 'cooling down' period of 15 days they have legislated. Note that we do not have any cooling-off period condition in the New Zealand Bill.

Jane says while the law hasn't changed on paper, the practice has. At first, mostly cancer patients and a few with terminal heart conditions requested it. "But over the last 12 years there's been a steady increase in numbers of those with chronic conditions wanting it—like those with diabetes, Parkinson's, neurological conditions, stuff that isn't necessarily terminal if people choose to have treatment."

The reasons for people choosing to use it is also very different to the original assumption that pain would be a motivational factor. "In 2019, 90 per cent of people in Oregon who requested assisted suicide did so because they didn't find life enjoyable. Fifty-nine per cent said they were requesting it because they were worried about being a burden on their families and caregivers. Pain or even just the fear of future pain was only mentioned by 33 per cent of people as a reason for wanting to die."

In Oregon a huge proportion of doctors refuse to prescribe lethal drugs, which means that 112 physicians wrote 290 prescriptions for lethal drugs in 2019. At least one doctor wrote 33 prescriptions that year. And the median length a doctor has known the patient is 14 weeks, with some doctors only knowing their patient for as little as one week.

"Studies have shown that while the safeguards claim to protect against mental illness, one in six people who have been prescribed lethal drugs suffered from clinical depression," Jane says.

There's some pretty hefty stats and observations so far. A pattern is emerging, and it isn't the one I hear from David Seymour.

We jump continents over to what some would say is the originator of euthanasia, or at least assisted suicide, to Switzerland. According to Article 115 of the Swiss criminal code of 1937, a person is allowed to assist in the suicide of another as long as the motive for doing so is not selfish.

Jane says the provision sat mostly untested until the 1990s with the rise of two prominent suicide promoters: Philip Nitschke from Australia, and Jack Kevorkian from the United States. "Nitschke [Philip] is a huge proponent of suicide. He believes anyone should be able to do it whenever they'd like, and he's dedicated much of his life to do just that."

> **"Studies have shown that while the safeguards claim to protect against mental illness, one in six people who have been prescribed lethal drugs suffered from clinical depression."**

Philip has written books and pamphlets about how to commit suicide and make it look like an accident. There was even a case in Australia of a man who cut all the pipes in his house and killed his wife, two disabled kids, and himself. They found he had accessed Philip's material and followed a plan that had been published.

Philip was instrumental in campaigning for euthanasia in the Northern Territories in Australia in the '90s. Technically the region was the first place to ever legalise it before being overturned by the Federal Government eight months after it was introduced. During that time, he euthanised four people.

In 1996 Philip helped set up an organisation called Exit International to enable people around the world to access information and support to commit suicide. Exit opened a clinic in Switzerland in 1997 to offer assisted suicide to Swiss residents and 'suicide tourists'. Other similar organisations followed including Dignitas and Lifecircle.

In 2017, Exit alone assisted 724 people to commit suicide.

Nearby neighbours, the Netherlands and Belgium, have had an underlying philosophy in their medical systems that there are some medical cases where there is just no good answer, Jane says. "You've given up all hope for a cure, nothing will help the patient get well, and they are suffering intensely—what will you do? Some doctors believed that the best course of action for these patients was to end their lives. These cases were taken to court and the courts routinely found doctors had committed no offence."

A new provision within this law allows euthanasia to be performed on a patient who has previously made a written request for death—even if, in their incapacitated state they now claim they don't wish to die.

In the early 2000s, both the Netherlands and Belgium made 'positive law' to codify the practice of assisted dying in their respective countries. The Netherlands, physician-assisted dying law was introduced in 2002, after being practised for decades.

Both euthanasia and assisted suicide are available for those experiencing unbearable suffering without the prospect of improvement. There is no requirement to be "terminally ill", nor is there any mandatory waiting period. A voluntary and well-considered request must be made and the patient must be fully informed and aware of their condition and options. A second opinion is needed and the euthanasia must be reported to one of the regional review committees.

Minors between 16 and 18 years of age can request euthanasia after consulting with their parents or guardians, but they do not need their permission. Children between 12 and 16 must have parental or guardian permission. A new provision within this law allows euthanasia to be performed on a patient who has previously made a written request for death—even if, in their incapacitated state they now claim they don't wish to die.

In one case a doctor disregarded judgments of a psychiatrist and performed euthanasia on a patient who was depressed and had reasonable options for effective treatment available.

And under a separate set of guidelines called the Groningen Protocol introduced in 2005, newborns can be euthanised if they are born with unbearable suffering, there is no alternative solution, and the parents, physician and an independent physician agree to the procedure. "As part of their review process, the review committees investigate cases in which, from the record provided to them by the doctor, they have concerns that the law has not been properly complied with," Jane says.

Jane pulls out a 2016 review. The committee had found 11 cases involving non-compliance with the law. In six of those cases the doctor did not comply with the criterion of due medical care. In three cases doctors did not properly consult with at least one other independent physician. In one case a doctor disregarded judgments of a psychiatrist and performed euthanasia on a patient who was depressed and had reasonable options for effective treatment available. And in another case a doctor performed involuntary euthanasia on an incompetent patient who insisted she did not want to die.

What? A doctor injected someone against their will? I investigate.

In 2019 a doctor accused of failing to verify consent before performing euthanasia on a dementia patient was cleared of any wrongdoing by a Dutch court.

A struggle ensued, and family members had to hold her down while the process was finished. The court ruled the doctor did not have to verify the current wish for death as the patient was demented and completely incapacitated.

The doctor's 74-year-old patient had written a statement after being diagnosed with Alzheimer's requesting euthanasia be given before she would need to be put in a care home. But she wanted to decide when the exact time was right. Before she was taken into care, the doctor decided that euthanasia should be administered based on her prior statement. This was confirmed by two separate doctors independently, and a date was set. The doctor put a sedative in her coffee and she lost consciousness. But the patient woke before the lethal injection was administered. A struggle ensued, and family members had to hold her down while the process was finished.

The court ruled the doctor did not have to verify the current wish for death as the patient was demented and completely incapacitated. "The use of premedication had been discussed with the family, and doctors were not negligent in this case. The proven offence is not punishable and the doctor is released from all legal proceedings," the court report stated. So the court basically nullified the second half of the woman's request, for her to consent to the injection at the time it was administered.

By 2010, Jane says, reports began showing that people were being euthanised for mental illness without any physical disease being present.

By 2012, 56 deaths of this nature were recorded. "In 2012, mobile euthanasia clinics began providing services to patients, including to those whose doctors had refused it as an option. There was no law change necessary for any of that to happen."

These cases and figures are a cause for concern as several elements of the EOLC Act are similar to the Netherlands' model—including the oversight mechanisms: SCENZ Group, the review committee and the registrar.

Next door, the Belgian law was introduced in 2002 for anyone 18 or older suffering from constant and unbearable physical or mental suffering that cannot be alleviated. There was never any terminal illness or foreseeable death requirement. In 2014, the law was amended to remove the age restriction, making it the most liberal law in the world. Children can now use it with a parent's permission. All medically-assisted deaths are reported to a Control and Evaluation Commission.

"The argument you hear from New Zealanders in reaction to this sort of information is the same as what the Canadians say—'They're just crazy Europeans; we won't get that far. Nothing like that will ever happen here'," Jane says.

In 2014, the law was amended to remove the age restriction, making it the most liberal law in the world. Children can now use it with a parent's permission.

But I can't help thinking that so many of us Kiwis want New Zealand to be considered a 'progressive' nation. We often hold up the Netherlands and Belgium in high regard with their tolerant stance on such issues. We cite their crime rates, their pro-choice, liberal stance. Our teenagers want to visit there… a country where there is 'no law' (or hardly any rules)... anything goes. Countries we admire.

Jane says for some people euthanasia has been attached to the idea of progress. "It's what progressive nations are doing… we're grown-ups, we can handle this." But she says no one can handle assisted dying.

She spent years speaking with MPs during her time in our country, sharing her research and trying to understand what their stance on euthanasia was. I don't understand how an MP can meet people like Jane and not come away with serious questions about the danger of introducing such a law.

"I've spoken to many, many politicians over the years—some personally and some in small groups," she says. "Those who are for euthanasia always fell into one of three categories: they had a personal experience with someone dying and they didn't like it, they have a fear of losing their abilities and dying in pain and suffering themselves, or they think they will never want to be euthanised but they can't deny someone who wants to use it.

"Nearly every one of them has a personal story. They watched a parent or grandparent die. A number of them say they wish they could have ended their suffering. Others have fears about their own death or ageing. They worry about getting a disability or a terminal illness, and all the things they think go with it… 'What if I can't feed myself or wipe my own bum?'. 'I don't want pain medicine', and 'I wouldn't be me anymore'.

"These are real fears, but they're not good grounds for making sweeping, complicated and dangerous laws."

As my time with Jane finishes I'm ready for a break. There's a lot to digest.

CHAPTER 17:

PROFESSOR THEO BOER

I couldn't find more of an insider than Professor Theo Boer. The father of two resides in the centre of Netherlands and has been immersed in the assisted dying culture of his home nation since the regime's origin.

Theo works 200km away from his home and commutes daily by train. Thankfully it's a fast train, he says. So I'm grateful for his time.

He is a qualified theologian and also studied bioethics and health law. He was recruited to one of the Netherlands' assisted dying regional review committees, its equivalent of the SCENZ Group, because of his reputation as a supportive critic to their law when it was introduced in 2002.

Theo says there was overwhelming support for euthanasia when it was introduced in the Netherlands and, as a democrat, he supported the majority decision. He was also in favour of bringing assisted dying into the open, to prevent the unofficial and illegal practice of doctors helping end the lives of terminally-ill patients, preferring it to happen with controls in place.

"I was invited by the former Minister of Justice as an ethicist to one of the five committees. I was sceptical of the law, I wasn't entirely in favour of its introduction but I was respectful of the compromise we reached with the law."

Theo would assess around 40 to 50 files and reports of euthanasia cases every month with his fellow committee members. And at first he was impressed with the way the law worked. "It seemed the law could contain the cases that were being presented."

But after a number of years, for reasons still unknown, the numbers went up. "The reasons people gave for choosing euthanasia widened; the pathologies increased. I became very uncomfortable about the situation."

The first major change seen was the tripling of the numbers of those using it. "It increased from 2,000 per year to 5,000." Then it went from just those with terminal cases, to chronic cases. "And then it changed from euthanasia being a last resort, towards patients using it as a right and a preferred way to die—a move to equate dignified dying and orchestrated dying."

So you're saying that while the law hasn't changed in the Netherlands its application has?

"The practice and interpretation of the law has definitely changed; it has evolved strongly."

In the Netherlands, Luxembourg and Belgium their law never included terminal illness as a requirement for assisted dying. It was just assumed most cases would take place in the context of terminal illness with the odd exception—because of this, Parliament did not restrict it, Theo says.

Originally around 97 per cent of the cases were for people within just days and weeks of their natural death. "It was the job of the review committees to ensure the law was being applied and interpreted correctly and that patients were in a hopeless situation. We were very strict on the interpretation. But it changed."

That cultural acceptance has paved the way to a law proposal Theo never thought could happen. "We have a proposal due to be tabled in the Netherlands about 'completed life'. The draft legislation proposes that anyone over 70 can have assisted dying irrespective of any medical necessity."

The proposal has been written from the prime minister's minor coalition partners D66, a liberal democratic party, and is aimed at providing suicide for elderly people "who consider their lives have been completed". It's targeted towards elderly people who have no sickness, but who are suffering from loneliness, bereavement and being disattached. And while originally there was an age limit of who could access it (which Theo references), two main political parties in support of the new law announced they will take the age criteria out altogether.

Initially, I caught myself in disbelief of what Theo was saying. This couldn't possibly be accurate. Firstly, what government would think this is a good idea? And secondly, why would anyone seriously consider their life has been 'complete'? But when I read more, I found myself shuddering at the reality that this could be on the near horizon.

In an interview with D66 MP Pia Dijkstra, Dutch newspaper *Algemeen Dagblad* (*AD*) reported that ministers were looking into the options for assisted suicide for people who are 'tired of life', but Pia said they weren't doing it quickly enough. "The Health Minister obviously senses the urgency less than I do. The very elderly who have had enough should be able to die when they choose to," Pia told the *AD*.

Theo says the proposal was supposed to be tabled the same week as our interview, but the COVID-19 lockdown had halted it. "We haven't heard anything. It loses momentum because society is focused on keeping people alive, our most vulnerable people, and keeping them from being affected. I hope it may cause a change in our focus."

The proposal followed a study published by the Dutch Ministry of Health which found there were a number of people aged 55 and over who, despite being in good health, "have a consistent and active desire to die".

It's of major concern for Theo as killing a human being should be an exception. "We shouldn't pretend that killing a human being whose natural life is not ended is normal. That is certainly not the view of Dutch doctors—they continue to stress that it is emotionally very burdensome to perform euthanasia."

"David Seymour is practically blind to any evidence. Seymour is categorically wrong. I know he is in favour of expanding the law—his commitment to limiting it to the terminally ill only is a stepping stone to expanding it to anyone who wants it and suffers unbearably."

David Seymour says that no law has changed in any jurisdiction that has it, and ours will be immovable.

"David Seymour is practically blind to any evidence. Seymour is categorically wrong. I know he is in favour of expanding the law—his commitment to limiting it to the terminally ill only is a stepping stone to expanding it to anyone who wants it and suffers unbearably."

I ask for proof. "Canada has just changed its law."

Theo is referring to a case in September 2019 where the Quebec Superior Court struck down a provision of their law which required someone's "natural death be reasonably foreseeable" before qualifying for medically-assisted dying.

In this particular case, the court ruled in favour of Nicole Gladu and Jean Truchon, both suffering from a serious degenerative disease, stating that the foreseeable death criteria is too restrictive and a violation of the Charter of Rights. Theo was a witness in that trial.

As a result the Federal Government introduced Bill C-7 to their parliamentary process on 24 February, 2020. The bill, among other things, removes the provision that restricts the procedure to those whose natural death is reasonably foreseeable. The Government has been given a deadline of 11 July, 2020 to amend the existing law.

Other changes being considered within that bill include removing the 'cooling off' period for those who are terminal, and introducing a 90-day wait period for those who aren't. Terminal patients will only need one witness, not two like currently required. That witness could be their healthcare provider or just a paid person. It also allows for advance directives for euthanasia.

As a result the Federal Government introduced Bill C-7 to their parliamentary process on 24 February, 2020. The bill, among other things, removes the provision that restricts the procedure to those whose natural death is reasonably foreseeable.

"All of this has happened before its five-year review period since the law's introduction lapsed," Theo says.

We don't have the same system of law as Canada, and our safeguards include terminal criteria. This couldn't happen to us… or could it?

"You will have a safeguard only as long as euthanasia activists will not appeal against it in court. I'm 100 per cent sure that David Seymour does not want to contain it within the six-month limit. He thinks there is a right for assisted dying for anyone suffering unbearably."

Theo predicts that within three years we will see someone contest the criteria in court saying it is unfair towards people with longer chronic illnesses. In that moment, David will argue society has evolved. "And in a way they are right. When it comes to unbearable suffering, frankly those who are frustrated the most are not the people with a couple of weeks left to live—they have access to excellent palliative care, great societal acceptance and sympathy. People who are truly suffering are those who have years or decades to live."

He says Parliament will be under duress to change the law. The

"Between the lines, particularly from the records, you could tell there was pressure from relatives."

process may be slightly different, but the pressure points remain true.

I'm interested in seeing whether Theo thinks the review committee model will stand up under pressure too. His understanding and perspective on how the committee worked in the Netherlands could be helpful.

Did you feel the regional review committees were objective enough to call people up to a standard?

"That's a hard question. We have a system where we scan doctors before they are approved to perform euthanasia—I think that is a more important process than the assessment of the cases. We assessed cases in hindsight.

"Were we sufficiently objective? We had five regions with five committees, each had three members, plus others involved. There were 45 of us involved in reviewing the practice and our own process. That was some guarantee of objectivity. What made me reverse my stance, though, was the committee's evolving view moving from being strict to becoming more liberal. The committees started encouraging people to explore what they called the 'full potential of euthanasia'. More and more, committees became supportive of it themselves."

As part of the committee process did you assess whether a patient was being coerced?

"We received a standard reporting form from the doctor and one of the standard questions was about whether there was any pressure on the side of the family members. The physician would say, 'No', or 'Perhaps, but I didn't see or recognise and I acted accordingly'. However, between the lines, particularly from the records, you could tell there was pressure from relatives.

"In several cases we had some clue there might have been some pressure. For example a written directive or advance directive written by the patient was signed with a signature which did not harmonise with the age and medical condition of the patient. We had a report where an elderly person of 87 had terminal cancer with a signature that was clearly not the patient's signature."

What did you do?

"We went back to the doctor and asked was this really the patient's signature? The doctor would say, 'Well it is as far as I know'.

"The point is, we were not police inspectors. If we asked a physician extra questions and the physician said, 'You can say rest assured', we had to leave it there."

So you perceived pressure in some cases but you couldn't prove it.

"It also depends on your definition of pressure. The hardest is not pressure from outside but the pressure that the patient has as a sponge, so to speak. The message a person sucks into himself and internalises so as to believe it. For example, there's continuous pressure from right-to-die societies that the only humane death is organised death. Anyone who is not having it will have a terrible death. This is pounding and pounding people. And in the end the patients themselves honestly think euthanasia is the best solution for them. In murder mystery films the most perfect murder is the one in which the victim themselves asked to be killed."

For example, there's continuous pressure from right-to-die societies that the only humane death is organised death. Anyone who is not having it will have a terrible death. "

Did you have any interesting cases come through that you had to inspect?

"I'm not allowed to talk about specific cases, but generally speaking there were two kinds of cases that were most problematic to me—one was the self-evidence. People with cancer, whose only focus was on euthanasia from the beginning. There was no alternative, no serious discussion about it because the patient had set their mind on this specific exit. Now we have excellent palliative care and the alternatives are well developed. A patient with terminal cancer doesn't need to be killed to have a humane death.

"The second example is the heartbreaking cases where a patient would have years or decades to live and there was an enormous despair for the patient. They were focused on having their death organised and there was a total absence of hope on the part of the caregivers, family members, and the patients themselves.

"I have known examples myself where people have been in despair for years and all of a sudden found their way up again and found new meaning in their lives. I found those cases heartbreaking from a humane perspective. I had serious doubts whether euthanasia was the solution there."

"The discussion, in my views is not about whether or not I have a right or not to kill myself. The discussion here is, I want others to provide my death. I don't think that is truly autonomous..."

Do you consider it a person's right to have this choice?

"There are people who spell autonomy with a capital I. If you and I would like to be dead we can be dead in half an hour. What this is about is not the right of a person to get killed, but to get help to get killed. If you are a truly autonomous person and you are sick of existing, then you should be free to do what you want unless you are in a proven psychiatric situation in which your mind isn't sound.

"The discussion, in my views is

not about whether or not I have a right or not to kill myself. The discussion here is, I want others to provide my death. I don't think that is truly autonomous: that is paradoxical."

So if this isn't about a person's rights, what is it about?

"In reality the discussion about euthanasia is about our inability to deal with despair. Inability to deal with tragedy and suffering. We need to explore what makes life so unbearable for people."

"In reality the discussion about euthanasia is about our inability to deal with despair. Inability to deal with tragedy and suffering. We need to explore what makes life so unbearable for people."

Theo gives an example to illustrate his point.

"Everyone remembers seeing the 9/11 scenes of people jumping out of the burning buildings after terrorists crashed planes into them. It doesn't make sense to say these people are not allowed to jump out of buildings; people are already jumping. However, it would also not make sense to say people have the right to jump… It's not the proper response because in either case there is a fire burning below them that is the real problem. That's why people are jumping.

"I think anyone in that situation would be happier if there was not a fire. Or if there was a staircase that could help them through the fire. The real problem is not whether these people want to die or not, the problem, is why are they suffering?"

And these people are vulnerable to assisted dying regimes?

"Euthanasia critics always point to the disabled, elderly and indigenous as vulnerable people. I think the true definition is anyone can be vulnerable psychologically, even the better off, even a person with a grand piano and woodblock floor and good income. True

"True vulnerability cannot be measured in terms of income or sickness but by having no psychological capacity to deal with suffering. It can happen to anyone."

vulnerability cannot be measured in terms of income or sickness but by having no psychological capacity to deal with suffering. It can happen to anyone."

A curious example of arbitrary law-making formulates in my head as I reflect on statements made about the illogical nature of making terminal illness a criteria...

I'd say most of us know what sibling rivalry looks like, and what's absolutely essential to the vocabulary of sibling law speech: "fairness".

"I want the big piece—why is he allowed that? It's not fair." I can hear the whining from younger years still ringing in my ears.

So I can easily imagine if one day I decided to hand out lollies to my eldest child, my youngest would be right at his heel with her arm outstretched and in an adorable yet demanding way, loudly proclaiming "Taaaaaaa" (she's one). If I say 'no' to her, we all know what follows... an almighty tantrum. In those moments as a parent we scramble for a justifiable reason why to deny one child over the other, hoping it will ease the sense of injustice.

In this case her brother is older, and we have a rule in our house: no lollies until you are two. But what happens if I had no good reason as to why I'm handing out lollies to one and not the other? How am I going to justify this to myself, let alone to the children?

And the older they get, the better they are at wrangling a just trial.

CHAPTER 18:

CASES

Researching international laws has led me into a forest of controversial claims. It's been mysterious and dark, and at times a little harrowing. But I've been strict in sifting, so stories I present are well documented. These cases have been reported by multiple mainstream media sources and associated governing bodies within the assisted dying practice.

The law in each jurisdiction varies, so comparisons will never be 100 per cent transferable, but key elements are. Cases have been selected to show how the law is being applied, interpreted, questioned and, in some cases, broken without consequence.

To note, no doctors have been charged with unlawful practice in any jurisdiction. Initially this was a comforting sign… but on closer inspection, it is extremely worrisome.

To note, no doctors have been charged with unlawful practice in any jurisdiction. Initially this was a comforting sign... but on closer inspection, it is extremely worrisome.

The Netherlands

In 2019 *The Observer* in the Netherlands reported that three deaths were being investigated by the public prosecution department for potentially breaching the law.

All were referred to the department by the Dutch regional euthanasia committees.

One involved an investigation into the case where a woman in her 70s with depression had been operated on for abdominal problems, when surgeons found evidence of lung cancer. She approached her doctor saying she was experiencing unbearable psychological suffering and wanted euthanasia. Her doctor's colleague took on the case, but, the review committee said, failed to obtain a second opinion from an independent psychiatrist, as is required.

The two other cases from 2017 involve a woman in her 60s with Alzheimer's who an independent consultant did not judge to be suffering badly enough, and another in her 80s with osteoarthritis and other problems who refused alternative treatment.

None of the doctors were charged.

Belgium

Three children under the age of 18 have been euthanised in Belgium. In 2014 the country amended its law on euthanasia to authorise doctors to administer it to a child of any age who is terminal, in unbearable suffering, and can make the request themselves. Children must be judged as having the mental capacity to make the decision, and must have parental consent.

During 2016 and 2017, a 17-year-old, an 11-year-old and a 9-year-old have been euthanised. The eldest was suffering from

During 2016 and 2017, a 17-year-old, an 11-year-old and a 9-year-old have been euthanised. The eldest was suffering from muscular dystrophy, the youngest had a brain tumour. And the 11-year-old suffered from cystic fibrosis.

muscular dystrophy, the youngest had a brain tumour. And the 11-year-old suffered from cystic fibrosis.

The Washington Post quoted a member of their euthanasia governing body, Dr Luc Proot, defending the cases saying, "I saw mental and physical suffering so overwhelming that I thought we did a good thing".

Interesting to note, in New Zealand our Attorney General released an analysis of the EOLC Bill to consider if it breached the Bill of Rights. As part of the review, it found that the legislation was discriminatory due to its age restriction in eligibility criteria. The Attorney-General recommended the age limit be reduced to 16 years old, or scrapped altogether.

Interesting to note, in New Zealand our Attorney General released an analysis of the EOLC Bill to consider if it breached the Bill of Rights. As part of the review, it found that the legislation was discriminatory due to its age restriction in eligibility criteria.

In 2020, three doctors were found not guilty of murder after euthanising a 38-year-old patient, despite family claiming the patient fell short of the serious and incurable illness requirement. The BBC reported the case, which involved Tine Nys being euthanised surrounded by her family in 2010.

Tine's sisters later argued her reason for seeking to end her life was because of a failed relationship, which did not meet the need for an incurable mental disorder in order to be euthanised. They said she suffered from depression and heroin addiction, and had previously tried to commit suicide several times. She had been diagnosed with autism two months before her death.

The manner in which the injection was given was also questioned as Tine's father was asked to hold the needle in his daughter's arm as the doctor had forgotten to bring plasters to secure it in place.

A 12-member jury delivered the verdict of not guilty. No explanation was given.

The lawyer of one of the doctors said a conviction would have established a dangerous precedent for professionals practising euthanasia. He said he and his peers had received dozens of letters from worried doctors who had halted euthanasia procedures for fear of legal consequences.

In 2013 *The Huffington Post* reported that a set of twins who were born deaf requested euthanasia after they discovered they might also become blind.

Marc and Eddy Verbessem, 45, were granted it after first being refused by their local hospital. Two years later they found another medical institution to administer the lethal injection. They were allowed its use on the grounds of "unbearable psychological suffering". Marc and Eddy's father and brother tried to talk them out of it, but to no avail.

The same doctor who euthanised Marc and Eddy also granted access to Nathan Verhelst, 44, who wanted it because his sex-change surgery did not work as desired. This caused him unbearable psychological suffering.

The doctor responsible was at the time the president of the euthanasia governing body in Belgium, Dr Wim Distelmans.

The same doctor is involved in a case taken to the European Court of Human Rights in 2019 in relation to the euthanasia case of Godelieva de Troyer, 64. The woman was euthanised for untreatable depression which was "largely the result of a break up with a man, but also due to her feelings of distance from her family," her son Tim claimed.

Tim has taken the case to court. He had only found out about his mother's death when the hospital called him the next day to pick up her body from the morgue.

Godelieva had a well-documented history of mental health problems. Her psychiatrist of more than 20 years confirmed she was not eligible.

The case is under investigation.

The same doctor who euthanised Marc and Eddy also granted access to Nathan Verhelst, 44, who wanted it because his sex-change surgery did not work as desired.

Canada

In 2017, *The Canadian Press* reported about a case involving 68-year-old woman Robyn Moro who had Parkinson's disease and received euthanasia. Canadian law at the time required a person's natural death to be "reasonably foreseeable".

Her doctor, Ellen Wiebe, had been cautious in considering Robyn's eligibility and denied her access at first. But in another precedent-setting case that was before the Ontario Superior Court around the same time, a ruling clarified that "reasonably foreseeable" didn't mean a person's illness must be terminal, their death imminent, or likely to occur within a specific time frame to meet requirements. So Ellen reconsidered and performed euthanasia on Robyn.

Ellen says the law is being unevenly applied across the country because of the ambiguity of the term "reasonably foreseeable". This criteria is currently being removed from the law altogether.

The family of a British Columbia man, Alan Nichols, who was euthanised in September 2019, are still looking for answers as to how he qualified for the procedure.

Alan, 61, had struggled with depression and showed no signs of facing an imminent demise, his family say. Yet he was euthanised despite pleas from his loved ones. Alan had a lifetime of struggle with depression and was admitted to hospital after being found dehydrated, weak and confused in his home weeks earlier, Canada's CTV News reported.

The family had been blocked from being involved in the process by Alan and therefore could not access any of the information around his death or eligibility. They were only permitted to attend his death.

At the hospital the family were told that two doctors had approved Alan's application for a medically-assisted death, and that a psychologist and psychiatrist were there to assess Alan's competence. The family weren't told on what grounds Alan had applied for euthanasia.

Alan's death certificate lists "medically-assisted death" as his immediate cause of death. Officials also listed three precursory causes connected to his death including a stroke, seizure disorder and "frailty". Other significant conditions not directly contributing to his death include the tumour he suffered as a child and the consequent insertion of a shunt to help relieve pressure on his brain.

The family have been told to request more information with the British Columbia Ministry of Health. They have hired a lawyer.

A Canadian hospice will be forced to close in February 2021 over its refusal to euthanise patients who requested an assisted death.

Fraser Health Authority, one of the six public healthcare authorities in the British Columbia province, pulled its funding from Irene Thomas Hospice. The authority also forbade the hospice from finding another partner to work with. The hospice received CA$1.4 million of its CA$3 million operating budget from Fraser Health, and funding for all 10 of its beds.

The authority intends to take over the Irene Thomas Hospice buildings and bring in medically assisted dying. The hospice buildings were constructed using CA$9 million of donations from community members.

Assisted dying is readily available at Delta Hospital, which is a one-minute drive from the Irene Thomas Hospice.

A Canadian hospice will be forced to close in February 2021 over its refusal to euthanise patients who requested an assisted death. Fraser Health Authority, one of the six public healthcare authorities in the British Columbia province, pulled its funding from Irene Thomas Hospice.

Quebec's College of Physicians released a letter to their Health Minister in 2018 raising concerns a lack of palliative care services may be forcing patients to choose assisted dying.

The group says Quebec is suffering from a shortage of specialised, palliative care doctors and uneven levels of service are being offered across the province. "Patients, failing to benefit from such care, could have had no other choice but to ask for medical aid in dying to end their days in dignity," the letter reads.

Group president Dr Charles Bernard said fewer physicians and medical professionals have chosen to specialise in palliative care over the last two years. "We are getting worried," Bernard told Canada's CBC News.

The Quebec Society for Palliative Care agreed. "When our patient tells us, 'Because I don't have enough help at home, because I'm stuck at a hospital, I'm going to request medical aid in dying,' doctors are uncomfortable," group president Dr Christiane Martel says.

A month later at a press conference held by a group of 10 Montreal-based physicians discussing the state of palliative care, Dr Pal Saba says fewer doctors had entered the field of palliative care since the law came into effect.

Group president Dr Charles Bernard said fewer physicians and medical professionals have chosen to specialise in palliative care over the last two years.

Speaking to Canada's CTV News the group also says the provincial government has provided them with little information on how they're managing the issue. "We were promised that there would be a plan for the development of palliative care in Quebec and the government commission asked for five years to develop this plan," Dr Laurence Normand-Rivest says. "We're in 2018, and for now, there's no plan."

Oregon

The Oregonian newspaper reported a case in 2005 of a man who had taken a lethal dose of medication in Oregon and woke up three days later.

David Prueitt, 42, was suffering from lung cancer and took the prescribed medication, but awoke asking, "What the hell happened? Why am I not dead?". He suffered no ill effects and was fully capable and competent… and surprised. He lived for two more weeks before dying of natural causes.

The Seattle Times reported David had taken the drug overdose prescribed, which had been mixed with apple sauce and water, in the presence of his wife, her mother, a friend and two Compassion in Dying volunteers. His wife had said he could barely raise the mug to his lips because he was so weak. Yet the drugs didn't work.

Prueitt told his wife he had been in the presence of God, and God had rejected his death by suicide and sent him back to live out his days and die a natural death.

The Oregonian newspaper reported a case in 2005 of a man who had taken a lethal dose of medication in Oregon and woke up three days later.

Oregon woman Barbara Wagner, 64, was refused funding for cancer treatment by her insurance company but in the same letter was told it would pay for assisted suicide medication.

America's ABC News reported in 2008 that Barbara had received bad news that the lung cancer which had been in remission had returned and would likely kill her. Her last hope was a US$4,000-a-month drug that her doctor prescribed for her, but the insurance company refused to pay.

Her oncologist had prescribed the drug Tarceva to slow the cancer's growth, giving her another four to six months to live. But under the insurance plan, she could only receive 'palliative' or comfort care, because the drug does not meet the 'five-year, 5 per cent rule'; that is, a 5 per cent survival rate after five years. What the Oregon Health Plan did agree to cover, however, were drugs for a physician-assisted death. Those drugs would cost about US$35 to $50.

The letter was recognised as a public relations blunder by the health plan spokesperson Jim Sellers. The organisation has since reviewed and changed its process, but the issue of pressure on physicians to control the cost of care is still present. The news article stated even those who support liberal death laws say Barbara's predicament is reflective of insurance attitudes nationwide.

A number of questionable cases have been reported by doctors themselves too, such as one by former associate professor of medicine at Oregon Health and Sciences University and practising physician Dr Charles Bentz.

"I was the primary care physician for an elderly gentleman for whom I made a diagnosis of melanoma and referred him to an oncologist. He was quite depressed because he was an avid outdoorsman—he loved to hike, he loved to be outdoors. He eventually asked this oncologist to give him physician-assisted suicide. His physician called and asked me to provide the second opinion as required by Oregon's law. I told my colleague that I objected and would not participate.

Oregon woman Barbara Wagner, 64, was refused funding for cancer treatment by her insurance company but in the same letter was told it would pay for assisted suicide medication.

"My concerns were ignored and two weeks later my patient was dead from an overdose of barbiturates prescribed by this oncologist. I later found out that a different physician had documented he was depressed. Instead of treating his depression, the oncologist gave him assisted suicide. I wondered and seriously doubted if this oncologist had addressed his suicidal tendencies.

"This is the real tragedy of assisted suicide in Oregon; instead of providing excellent care, my patient's life was cut short by a physician who did not address the issues underlying his suicidality."

> **"My concerns were ignored and two weeks later my patient was dead from an overdose of barbiturates prescribed by this oncologist. I later found out that a different physician had documented he was depressed. Instead of treating his depression, the oncologist gave him assisted suicide."**

Nevada physician Brian Callister has spoken out about two patients who were denied life-saving treatments by insurance companies refusing to pay, but offering assisted suicide as an alternative.

Brian attempted to transfer two of his patients to California and Oregon in 2017 for procedures not performed at his hospital. Representatives from two insurance companies denied transfer requests; in both cases medical insurance directors asked if assisted suicide would be considered instead.

CHAPTER 19:

DAVID SEYMOUR MP

David Seymour has been the driving force behind the EOLC Act. Sure, he's inherited a momentum from those that have gone before, but he's also punted it along the political process and in the public arena like no one else.

So when there was a chance to interview him after an End-of-Life Choice Society meeting, I took it. I'm glad to have caught him relaxed, away from the media headlights and rabid debating chambers of Parliament.

My initial impression was surprising. I hadn't really expected him to be around the same height and age as me, or to find him relatable and humorous, albeit a little smarmy. I think politics and the glaring spotlight of live cameras ages people. I don't envy a politician's job at all and have a real respect for the enormity of their task and the challenge of job security hinging on public popularity. It's not comfortable.

I appreciate his willingness to take an impromptu interview as I pullout the voice recorder and we go 'on the record'. I ask David why he chose to enter the EOLC Bill into the ballot box.

"I stood for Parliament to improve New Zealand's laws. I found myself as a sole MP [in my Party] with very few options for doing that. And I saw I could make a huge difference here because people do suffer, and we want a compassionate society. I think people suffering at the end of their life should have the freedom to make that choice.

"I saw an opportunity to give that choice. And I'm pleased I'm halfway to delivering it. As Chris Bishop National Party MP said in his third reading, it will make us a more humane and compassionate society. That is the job of a politician."

Every politician has owned up to their own personal motivational story in this—surely David has one too?

"I don't have a particular personal dog in this fight. Some people think it's because my mum died when I was relatively young. It's true, she did. But she died very comfortably in a hospice and I'm grateful for that. She wouldn't have used this law—I personally think she would have supported it, though."

David says most people support assisted dying laws. "If you look at the desire for this law change it's been pretty consistent. If you talk to Jessica Young, who did her PhD on this [*Perspectives on assisted dying from people approaching the end of life*] at Otago University, she found that the support hadn't changed in 20 years. Jessica analysed every poll back to 2002 and averaged them out at 68 per cent in favour."

David says what has changed over time is the fact that other countries have introduced similar laws. "When Michael Laws introduced his bill in '95 no other country had legalised it. By 2003 Belgium, Oregon and the Netherlands had it. You could no longer say 'this is crazy; it doesn't work'. But you could still say it's a new thing. Then the Lecretia Seales case catalysed it, like Brittany Maynard did in California. I mean, having an attractive, articulate woman who had done everything right in her life and had this unfortunate illness and just wanted to choose—that's a pretty compelling reason why to support it. She's reasonable, not crazy... That helped as well.

"Then it took two years to get my Bill drawn—that was just random luck."

Seeing other countries trial the laws and processes has made it feel a little less risky, but it isn't all smooth sailing. I ask David if he thinks the laws are holding up.

"People say these terrible things happen in other countries that have introduced the law," David says firmly. "But they just don't."

I can't quite let that slide totally uncontested. So I ask him if he has heard about the case of the 74-year-old dementia patient who was euthanised against her request.

"That's probably one case I would spend some time on. But first of all, it's not relevant to New Zealand because we don't allow advance directives so we wouldn't have that situation. What appeared to have happened in her case is throughout her life she said that she wanted it. But in the end she lost her mind and said 'no'. But her son said, 'Come on, you've told us your whole life…'

"Now I think they did the wrong thing legally and morally. But you can understand why they would think they were doing the right thing. That's why we didn't put advance directives in our law. In any case, the fact we know about that case, and it was tried through the courts, shows you the law is working as it should."

I can't help noticing some contradiction in this explanation. I follow David's point that the case isn't directly relevant as our law won't allow for advance directives. And the fact the case was flagged and investigated shows there is some scrutiny in the processing. But David himself acknowledges it wasn't legally good or morally sound. Yet no one got prosecuted or held to account. Isn't that a "terrible thing" that "just doesn't" happen? Is the law actually doing what it claims?

David says no law is perfect. "We have lots of laws against all sorts of things that people break. That's not to say the law doesn't work. Actually almost no one breaks this law, but when it is [broken], it's dealt with properly.

"I always urge people to be cautious when you hear these stories. People say there are death ambulances driving around the Netherlands picking up grandmas. It's bullsh*t."

I ask him if there are other major rumours that jump out as misinformation.

"If you've ever been in a debating society there are people who are just sh*ts. They bring up stuff they know they don't really believe but it casts doubt on the debate. It muddies the water enough. It's something you would expect from lawyers or politicians."

An example of some mud? "Undetectable coercion. Some say, what if there is undetectable coercion operating? Well I'd say, 'F*ck, you wouldn't know, would you?' But actually, funnily enough, we can know."

I ask David what he thinks about the debate surrounding the terminology of a doctor 'having to do their best' as a poor standard.

"At some point you've got to be honest about the real motivation [of the opposition]. You've got a group of people that believe God gives you life and it's God's choice to take it away. If a whole lot of people say, 'No, that's bullsh*t; we're going to make a choice for ourselves', that undermines everything those people believe and they just can't handle it."

"There are other areas where doctors just have to do their best to achieve something. But I'd say you have to look at who uses the law overseas—if coercion was a problem you would see people of low education using it, people susceptible to being pushed around. But it's actually the opposite—people who are educated, have better access to palliative care, people who have more assertive personality traits.

"It makes perfect sense—the whole thing is bureaucratic. You've got to be willing to push your way through it to get it. If there was a whole bunch of vulnerable people being steered into it I obviously wouldn't be doing this."

David says if the application process is quite rigorous it will be the articulate and well-resourced people willing to fight through the red tape to use it. "At some point you've got to be honest about the real motivation [of the opposition]. You've got a group of people that believe God gives you life and it's God's choice to take it away. If a whole lot of people say, 'No, that's bullsh*t; we're going to make a choice for ourselves', that undermines everything those people believe and they just can't handle it. They will do and say just about anything to undermine it… which is interesting because they are breaking a lot of other religious edicts along the way, such as, 'don't lie'.

Firstly, I consider disqualifying a person's opinion based on a religious belief is discriminatory. And secondly, no one has spoken of any religious concern as a motivational factor to me.

"Of course the majority of people of faith are in favour of this law—we know this by polling."

David says in the census half of New Zealanders profess to having a Christian faith, and more than half of Kiwis are in favour of assisted dying as a concept.

David then goes on to list a number of organisations and individuals who have spoken out about the Act and their religious affiliation, in an accusing and agitated tone. Some of them include people who I have interviewed. "You scratch the surface, all of them; you can draw a straight line back... Even the disability groups; if you scratch the surface... you try and find an opponent of any serious scale who's not religiously motivated."

I couldn't help but feel like I was being let inside a conspiracy theory, one that David was personally frustrated by.

Firstly, I consider disqualifying a person's opinion based on a religious belief is discriminatory. And secondly, no one has spoken of any religious concern as a motivational factor to me.

As he's opened the gate, I ask David what his religious upbringing was.

"I'm a baptised Presbyterian," he jokes. "Only because my mum was so mortified at having a boy she realised it was the last chance to put me in a dress [for baptism]."

We laugh, but I persist. Were you raised Presbyterian? What's your story?

"I just believe in a free society. My maxim is, 'If you're not hurting anyone else, then you can do whatever you want.' I'm so busy running my own life I don't have time to judge other people. Wouldn't it be a much nicer, prosperous, humane place if we would stop interfering with other people's business?"

Isn't that a little ironic coming from a politician whose job it is to write a law for everybody?

"That's what I love about it. It's a counter-intuitive challenge. Everybody else is trying to win power so they can wield it against other people, but I'm trying to win it so I can not use it. Much harder, but isn't it a great challenge?"

So, what is the purpose of the law in our country then?

"There's a legitimate role for the government in a free society to regulate market failures. That's where everybody does their best but collectively the result is bad."

Our interview comes to a finish as society members bump past us on their way out, wanting to shake David's hand and encourage him.

David's done a brilliant job at succinctly packaging the law... a bit of a Pandora's box tightly wrapped and neatly tied. It looks real pretty. And he's sticking to it.

CHAPTER 20:

REV. JOHN FOX

"Personal Account

If religion really is the root of all evil when it comes to the opposition of assisted dying then Reverend John Fox would be a henchman...

Meet the Reverend John Fox. Direct. Intelligent. Busy. And disabled. John is a trustee at Elevate Christian Disability Trust, an ordained Anglican minister and is a staunch disability advocate. In his spare time he visits elderly parish members for a cup of tea to keep them company, then goes home and plays Xbox. There's no way he's a henchman.

I speak with him over Skype at his home in Christchurch. John's in his 30s with his short dark brown hair, thinly-framed rectangular glasses, and friendly demeanour keeping him youthful.

John was born with spastic hemiplegia, a form of cerebral palsy, after oxygen deprivation damaged his motor neurons at birth. He has an incurable medical condition that involves disability and, in his case, a decline in mobility as an adult. His earliest memory is of pain. When he was four and his Achilles tendon was cut in order to lengthen it.

John vividly remembers screaming when his foot was pushed down to flatten it. "Doctors tried to explain to me what was happening but I was just too young to understand."

This was only the first time of many when John felt vulnerable in a medical setting. In 2005 a bout of glandular fever caused Chronic Fatigue Syndrome, which affected his nervous system and resulted in two episodes of significant decline in mobility. And while he has faced many battles John has also succeeded in many achievements, one among other things was acquiring a PhD.

So what does John think about this Act?

"I think it's iniquitous. For a start, it proceeds from a profound fear of disability. I've talked to maybe 40 MPs personally. Every single one has brought up the basic idea that they wouldn't want to be stuck having their bum or drool being wiped by another person, and not being independent. That mentality, from a disabled person's perspective, basically says 'better dead than you'.

"I've talked to maybe 40 MPs personally. Every single one has brought up the basic idea that they wouldn't want to be stuck having their bum or drool being wiped by another person, and not being independent. That mentality, from a disabled person's perspective, basically says 'better dead than you'."

"It's saying everyone who is dependent on someone—all the elderly, the disabled, the sick—are undignified. The assumption seems to be that being able-bodied and not dependent on anyone is the best option. Or to become dependent or disabled takes away from your humanity. I'm not going to accept that assumption.

"There is a message which is being sent by this Act to disabled people by saying there is a moment at which you don't count... a moment where your life is no longer valuable. That worries me. If you want to say there is a moment, you have to make a statement which categorises it. Is it when you are in terrible pain? Well I'm in pain right now. Is it the quality of life? Someone loses independence? What does that mean for elderly people or quadriplegics? Is it that someone is going to die? Well we are all going to. When does a request for suicide become legitimised?"

John says he doesn't see any difference between assisted dying and suicide. "I know people say they are different, but I have seen no argument to substantiate this. So I call it what it is."

John says he doesn't see any difference between assisted dying and suicide. "I know people say they are different, but I have seen no argument to substantiate this. So I call it what it is."

John meets and speaks with vulnerable people every day, in his role at Elevate, a chaplain in a rest home, and as a Minister. One of his big concerns is the EOLC Act enables suicide. "I'm very uneasy about the Act as I don't believe in enabling suicide. I don't like the idea that disability or illness is 'less than', and there are lives we don't want to protect or aren't worth protecting."

He says it's profound to him that we are considering a law that in certain circumstances would allow us to just accept someone's desire to die prematurely. "When an able-bodied person comes to you and says they want to die, you ask 'Why?'. But when someone who is terminally ill comes, you say it is 'OK'."

He says in every situation where someone is requesting death they should be questioned and helped. "For example, what's the context? What medication are you on?... You do a holistic analysis as to why someone is experiencing this. You help them find meaning and purpose again, help them adjust their medication… but in this case, if the law passes you just accept a suicide request.

"People who want to commit suicide aren't seeing the rest of their lives, the possibilities, the help to get them out of the rut. It's solidarity and kindness to help people in these moments—whether they are dying or not.

"The worst thing is when someone doesn't feel their value. There does come a moment when you don't feel that and other people have to hold it for you. That's what our society should be doing with people suffering."

Having access to euthanasia and assisted suicide is creating a temptation for the vulnerable, especially for those at the severe end of disability.

"At Elevate we are very well aware—we take care of people from the mild end through to motor neuron disease, the really nasty things. We spend quite a lot of time counselling people who have become disabled, reframing the feeling that if you become disabled your life is over. While a certain kind of life is over, there are lots of people who love you. It's like bereavement to adjust to those sorts of changes. It can take between 8 and 10 years to adapt. Some clearly do it quicker, some need support, and others need ongoing help. We are having to work with people in really dark spaces dealing with chronic pain. There are many vulnerable moments.

"When I was at the pain clinic one of the things they asked was how many times have I wanted to kill myself. I asked my pain team how many people come to the clinic who are suicidal—they said about half, especially if someone has become disabled. Pain is a risk factor for suicide; so is disability."

But you aren't eligible for assisted dying if you are merely disabled or old.

"Legal advice I have received has been that this Act is really badly written; it's ludicrously broad. And yes, I probably could be eligible.

We asked the Oregon Department of Health what they define as terminal in the United States. They said 'anything that can kill you in six months'. So does diabetes count if you don't take your medication? 'Yes'. It could be easy for some of us who are disabled to cross over into the terminal category if we wanted to. We know from other jurisdictions that already have this, the category will get broader in practice."

Then there's the risks to the Act's application?

"I know how the medical system works, I know what pain is, and I know how many people make mistakes. I know the reality of bureaucracy and the district health board—even just with ordinary things like getting your meds right, getting you to appointments and getting a specialist. Cerebral palsy is quite well known and yet I still catch doctors having to look up what my illness actually is. And I know how vulnerable I feel as part of that system. I know how radically vulnerable the whole thing is, before you even put a question of death on it. There are bound to be mistakes and difficulties. There are bound to be inconsistencies of care in any system.

"I know how radically vulnerable the whole thing is, before you even put a question of death on it. There are bound to be mistakes and difficulties."

"I'm still not convinced the checks and balances are appropriate. Euthanasia prosecutions in other jurisdictions are rare because it's hard to get good information. The 'good faith' clause says that provided you are trying to give effect to someone's wishes or at least you thought you were, you are protected. It's hard to get prosecutable facts when your chief witness is dead."

He worries about those who are disabled and have communication difficulties. "I've worked with some and it's hard to know whether they want broccoli or cauliflower… It's going to be extremely hard to know what their wishes are and if the family can sign the paper for you. How are we going to know they weren't coerced? There's still very weak accountability for the doctors involved in this; the penalty a doctor can receive if they make a mistake is $10,000. David Seymour said that is primarily just a slap on the hand for not filling in the form correctly.

"There's a number of really problematic elements in terms of how it will work that haven't been addressed."

Is it merely a religious stance John has taken on the issue? He says he was opposed to the Act before he was ordained. "But the religious perspective says we are all valuable because we are made in the image of God and we are to protect the vulnerable because they can't protect themselves. That's a common belief in a number of religions. And you don't even have to be religious to believe that."

> **"There's still very weak accountability for the doctors involved in this; the penalty a doctor can receive if they make a mistake is $10,000. David Seymour said that is primarily just a slap on the hand for not filling in the form correctly."**

His role as a priest means he has witnessed 'normal' death and painful death a number of times. "Most of us really don't know what normal death looks like. In one of her speeches MP Nikki Kaye said it's her philosophical position that no one should be in pain… does she not live in the world with the rest of us? There comes a moment in life when awful things happen. I'm not meaning to knock her, but if you expect life to be that easy you are going to be disappointed and frightened of death. People say they saw a grandparent die and it was hard and traumatic… well of course it was—that's part of dying. Every death looks uniquely terrible. Many cultures around the world have a cultural category for dying, an accepted way of doing it.

"There are genuinely hard cases and failures and patchiness in services. But a lot of the way people die and a lot of dignity they receive in their death depends on how other people around them carry them."

"We are undermining some key things which make sure vulnerable people are safe. We are establishing a rule that will put a whole bunch of vulnerable people under pressure to justify the value of their lives."

If John could speak to all those with disabilities in New Zealand facing this vote: "I would say I love you. I would say lots of people love you. Your life is valuable and necessary and equal. Your pain is important and difficult but also think about how this is going to affect others and the care and services we will have in the long term.

"I'd ask people to think how it would feel to deliver euthanasia. We should not expect doctors to do it. We are undermining some key things which make sure vulnerable people are safe. We are establishing a rule that will put a whole bunch of vulnerable people under pressure to justify the value of their lives. I would ask other disabled people and other New Zealanders to remember their value and vote accordingly."

While walking with the kids to the beach, I am starting to recognise that my thoughts towards others are changing. There are older people swimming in the cooling autumn waters. Their wrinkles and hobbles are taking on new meaning. I can walk to the beach from my house with no personal health restrictions; I'm free to make myriads of independent choices every day. And I'm starting to recognise this is not a regular occurrence for everyone in our community: it's a privilege and I've taken it for granted.

Sometimes it takes a confrontation from someone in a different situation that wakes you up. Sometimes it's when things get stripped away that you realise what you had. But I think it's always being thankful that can help inoculate you against entitlement.

It's the thankfulness that Vicki, Claire, Huhana, Paula and John carry to be alive that has helped them flourish.

SECTION 6:

RELIGIOUS RESPONSES

There is a claim that all opposition to assisted dying derives from religious roots. Not only has that statement been offered in a discriminatory tone, but it also just hasn't measured up. Only five to 10 per cent of submissions to the Select Committee contained religious arguments. And I've actually had to vigorously pursue religious leaders to specifically get their religious take.

What is consistent, though, is that a huge number of religious organisations made submissions based on concerns around key elements of the EOLC Act, particularly, thoughts around what true compassion means and the protection of human life being a fundamental cornerstone of society. Leaders from Catholic, Baptist, Presbyterian, Anglican and Lutheran churches, The Salvation Army, Muslim groups and associations, and even a Buddhist group contributed.

I've cornered a Catholic, Protestant and a Muslim leader for comment.

CHAPTER 21:

DR JOHN KLEINSMAN

Some interviews seem to have a running start, like the person is an idling Ferrari waiting for the lightest touch of the accelerator to elicit a monumental response. Others feel a bit more like a diesel engine, needing a decent warm-up and a good rev first. The Catholic Nathaniel Centre's John Kleinsman is one of the latter.

Don't get me wrong: he is excellent at communicating, he's got a good grip on the issues and carries a decent portion of wisdom. I like him. But it's hard to know where to start. Maybe it's a result of the enormity of the task. Maybe we need a second coffee. In fairness, I'm not used to having to warm up any engine when it comes to the issue.

John Kleinsman's got a PhD in science and a masters in theology and has been working at the centre which is a hub for bioethics research for 20 years, 10 of which as director. The centre's essentially an agency of the New Zealand Catholic Bishops Conference. They advise bishops for their own deliberation, sometimes speak for them in a public capacity and help formulate 'official statements' like the submission they made to the Justice Select Committee on the EOLC Act.

I approached John for an interview to get a Catholic perspective on the issue. His response isn't exactly what I expected.

"This question of how to vote isn't specifically a religious one. I've heard religious arguments for and against the issue of assisted dying. But our position is first and foremost informed by the concern we have about the impact it will have on vulnerable New Zealanders. Religions bring a message of love and inclusion and care of vulnerable people."

John is also forward in letting me know he personally is opposed to it, his opinion based on what he has researched and his work. "I would remain opposed even if the Pope changed his mind—which I don't think he will."

From a Catholic perspective, is this issue black and white?

"Catholic teaching is very clear on this; there really isn't much wriggle room. But it's a teaching based on the impact and consequences."

How does the Bible weigh into the Catholic perspective? Are there any particular passages that say assisted dying is 'sin'?

"We have a deep and long standing philosophical and theological tradition we work out of. The scriptures [the Bible] are absolutely critical in terms of our understanding of revelation and informing our views on different things. But when you come to specific scriptures, they don't always give you clear responses to these sorts of questions. There is no body of teaching per se that talks about some of these issues... like some of the ethical questions around genetic modification and artificial reproductive technologies. So the challenge for me is to apply key principles and work out this vision of human flourishing so we can navigate our way through."

One of these principles is approaching the issue from an 'us' perspective. To illustrate this John tells me about a meeting he attended three years ago in the lead up to the 2017 General Elections. Candidates were asked their opinion on a number of issues, including assisted dying. "A candidate stood and identified himself as Catholic and said 'The way I think about it is, how would I feel living in the shoes of a person with cancer?'."

John points out that the man usually started his sentences with 'the way I think'… "That is a very self-referential view. The Catholic approach would be an another-referential perspective. It's not that we ignore the person's beliefs, but it is not where we start. Questions like 'Will someone be margalised?', 'What is the impact on others?',

'What is the intergenerational dynamic?' must be at the forefront of consideration. While we don't deny personal choice, we start from a perspective that we are relational humans who live with other people. The idea that we are all individual, autonomous people is very different to the authentic Catholic approach."

John says in applying that approach to the EOLC Act we would have to consider the society we live in. "There are rising rates of elder abuse, rising rates of older people finding themselves socially isolated, a functionalist approach to understanding and valuing human life… we are living in a very ableist and ageist time. When you put that all together it's absolutely clear from a Catholic perspective this is something that is far too dangerous to introduce. You couldn't do it safely in the current context."

"We are living in a very ableist and ageist time. When you put that all together it's absolutely clear from a Catholic perspective this is something that is far too dangerous to introduce. You couldn't do it safely in the current context."

The ableism and ageism have created a systemic coercion that is too hard to protect people from, John says. "The NZMA [New Zealand Medical Association] and doctors have made it very clear they would struggle to detect overt pressure such as psychological abuse, but I think the more dangerous form is the idea that somehow if you become dependent on others because you are elderly, disabled or sick, you are a burden.

"An MP said to me the new narrative is, 'The brave thing is not to be a burden'. If you compare society today to 20 years ago, we just aren't in the same position to care for needy members as we were then. It's not a moral issue, it's just a fact. Families are smaller and more geographically spread out; if you live in one of the big cities as a couple, both partners need to work to pay for the basics. We talk a lot about being asset rich and time poor. People don't have time to care for those with needs and somehow as a society we have this idea that being a burden is something we need to avoid."

The sense of being a burden is close to home for John.

"I saw the pressure in my own dad as he was dying," he says. "A sense of somehow 'if I am being a burden I don't have a right to be here'.

"We saw it emerge in conversations around COVID-19. When you are alert to it, you see it everywhere. We talk about the 'grey tsunami'—a phrase used a lot to describe baby boomers reaching retirement age. A tsunami is one of the most destructive forces we know. Listen to our language, our attitudes.

"We talk about the 'grey tsunami'—a phrase used a lot to describe baby boomers reaching retirement age. A tsunami is one of the most destructive forces we know. Listen to our language, our attitudes."

"A longitudinal study out of Auckland showed more than 54 per cent of people aged 65 or older describe themselves as incredibly lonely."

John says this undercurrent leaves people feeling they have to justify the right to live. "The 'right to die' becomes a 'duty to die'. I see it as a powerful argument. It represents one of the biggest but least talked about issues."

This pressure was something John's own father carried in his last months before death. "I got to see how vulnerable Dad was before he died last year [in 2019]. Before the third reading, this Act included the grievous or irremediable suffering criteria and I was acutely aware my dad would have qualified for it. In his journey I saw how fragile he was day-to-day, his whole outlook on life went up and down. And I saw how easily he could be convinced his life wasn't worth living. He was actually depressed.

"It occurred to me how easy, in that context, it would have been for him to say, 'This is my life and this is what I want to do' [apply for assisted dying]."

"The 'right to die' becomes a 'duty to die'. I see it as a powerful argument. It represents one of the biggest but least talked about issues."

For John it highlighted the need for him to tell his dad how much he mattered and how much he was loved. "We talked about assisted dying and the law; Dad put a submission in against it himself. But there were times where he said he could understand why some would want it."

John says his dad wanted to die at home. "In the end we were all with him. Not every day was easy, but we had lots of laughs along the way; lots of beautiful things happened. A lot of sad things too. It wasn't easy, but it was a wonderful journey. For him, knowing that we were there and he wasn't alone was pivotal. He relaxed into it almost.

"The fear is real, but we've got ways of dealing with it… it's called caring."

David Seymour says the EOLC Act offers compassion by providing a choice which is within a law that is safe and secure.

"I absolutely refute that. It isn't safe, and its eligibility criteria will change. Evidence from overseas shows the way the law has been interpreted changes and in some jurisdictions now allows for people with dementia, for children, and people with mental illness like depression."

John is referring to the Netherlands and Belgium.

"And it makes sense for it to change... why would you give choice to a certain number of suffering people and not others? What about all those people who have neuro-degenerative diseases who have several years to live? They are the ones who have the strongest case for it. That's not fair. It's an irrational argument; it's an arbitrary line.

"David Seymour has said himself on numerous occasions he tightened the eligibility to get the Bill through. That's smart politics. And it's nothing more than politics. It can't hold and it won't hold. The only way you can justify or agree to any form of assisted dying is to buy into the principle that some lives are less worth living than others. You cannot escape that."

John was instrumental in writing a submission on the EOLC Bill to the Justice Select Committee on behalf of the Nathaniel Centre. He was also involved in penning a collaborative open letter to MPs about the Bill from a group of high-level religious representatives including the president of the New Zealand Catholic Bishops Conference, the national leader of the Baptist Churches, the territorial commander of The Salvation Army, a number of bishops from the Anglican Diocese, and the bishop of the Lutheran Church.

"The only way you can justify or agree to any form of assisted dying is to buy into the principle that some lives are less worth living than others. You cannot escape that."

Both of those documents listed a number of 'grave' concerns primarily from an ethical, philosophical and practical perspective. It's fair to say the general religious stance is in opposition to the Act and assisted dying. Religious leaders stated they speak from their extensive experience of actively caring for the dying and their family.

"We know the need for and effectiveness of holistic and compassionate end-of-life palliative care. But high-quality palliative care is not yet equitably accessible throughout New Zealand and until it is, there is a strong likelihood that New Zealanders will also choose assisted death because of a lack of other meaningful choices. In such a context, there is the real risk that people in lower socio-economic groups will find themselves being channelled unnecessarily and unjustly towards a premature death."

John says the irony of the 'choice' argument is that the law only mandates one choice. There is no mandate of good palliative care being offered.

"We know palliative care is not easily accessible by all and the quality of end-of-life care around New Zealand differs greatly… If you live somewhere where you don't have access to good palliative care, what sort of choice is there really? I agree there is a problem in that too many are suffering, but is assisted dying the best, most caring response we can come up with? It is not the answer."

"I agree there is a problem in that too many are suffering, but is assisted dying the best, most caring response we can come up with? It is not the answer."

Among concerns raised about the Act is the significant impact it will have on our legal system, John says. "In the current law everybody is equal and the starting assumption is we should never kill another person. We accept there are rare circumstances where one person could kill a person. The clearest example is killing in self-defence… but the starting point is that this should never happen. In those sorts of circumstances, which are rare and exceptional, the justice system will test that. So every single case is tested and every death is investigated under the current criminal system.

"The onus is on the person who killed somebody to prove they acted proportionately. The law assumes everybody deserves to live."

But with the introduction of a law like the EOLC Act, the starting point will shift.

"The law will have to treat some people differently on the basis of their ability [health]. And while David Seymour says he's taken disability out of the picture, in fact it's all about disability and functionalism. Intentional death is no longer going to be an exceptional death. There will be a whole cohort of people who can be killed and there will be no investigation or examination of the circumstances in which that death happened."

"There will be a whole cohort of people who can be killed and there will be no investigation or examination of the circumstances in which that death happened."

I asked why he thinks us Kiwis are so unaware or not engaged in this issue if it's fundamentally going to change the fabric of our law.

"I don't know, I've scratched my head over that. I think we've grown up in a neoliberal fishbowl; it's the water we're swimming in. The 'choice' and 'individualism' are important parts of the narrative that we use to make sense of the world in which we live. Within that particular narrative assisted dying does make sense. To me, it's a very impoverished narrative.

"It's hard to unpack that: it's a complex argument. And the choice argument appeals; it provides what looks like a very neat cut-through... 'You know if you don't want it, John, that's fine—but why deny my choice?'

"It's naive because our choice impacts other people, we don't make it in isolation and its impact isn't only on us. With the work I do, I try to teach people to look at their underlying narrative. What are the consequences of buying into that narrative?

"It's much easier to wheel a terminally-ill person onto the stage than to wheel a terminally-ill society… It's easier to argue in favour than against because a lot of the arguments against it are in a sense more philosophical. It's about consequences that haven't yet happened; about facts we don't want to accept."

I come away from the time with John considering his last thoughts. What narrative am I living in? It's fairly difficult to assess our own lens of perception on life. And it's something we hardly ever do. The reason we have our lens in the first place is because of our own experiences and beliefs. They are pretty foundational elements that influence our choices every day, including our thoughts around assisted dying. To consider a lens properly we would have to hold our core values lightly.

But in a world where self-awareness is king, we still aren't very good at perceiving our own biases, or measuring our own measuring stick. Our own truth really has become the truth.

But in a world where self-awareness is king, we still aren't very good at perceiving our own biases, or measuring our own measuring stick. Our own truth really has become the truth.

There's actually a word for that. It's called relativism—a philosophical position that morals are created from subjectivity. Whether something is right or wrong is determined by the norms of the society we live in. Relativism would say, 'My right doesn't have to be your right. And quite frankly, you can't tell me what my right or wrong is—only I can do that.' I wonder how much the virtue of autonomy has grown out of this soil.

One of the only ways I know how to recognise my own perception is by comparing it to something else. We need each other to be able to do that.

Catholicism would say the only absolute point of comparison is the Bible. And for those who discount religion altogether, I wonder where their moral compass finds its bearing? True north has to be an unchangeable location, otherwise the compass is going to direct us all over the show.

CHAPTER 22:

PROFESSOR DAVID RICHMOND

Being bound to the borders of Summerset retirement village in Ellerslie during COVID-19 level-four lockdown doesn't stop Professor David Richmond from putting forward his thoughts on assisted dying—at least not via a phone interview.

Village residents can't go outside the gate and shopping has to be done for them. His description sounds almost a little prison-like in my opinion, but David says it isn't too bad. While they can't use the indoor pool and spa, or the bowling green, he is keeping himself busy with projects. That's no surprise considering David's background.

A retired doctor, David served as the chair of the Auckland Hospital Research Ethics Committee, and was the inaugural professor of geriatric medicine at the University of Auckland. He's also been the Dean of Theology at that university and stood in national positions within the Baptist Churches of Aotearoa. So, he can bring a multi disciplinary take on the issues. And although he is a bit of a veteran on the topic, becoming involved in the early 2000s, he says he has been sidelined for much of the more recent discussions. But I've called him 'off the benches' to help me understand why assisted dying is largely opposed in Christian circles.

David says Christians should be compelled to discover as much as possible about the Act, learn what they can about the effects of it on communities that have already legalised it, and search scriptures for guidance about the morality of it. And if they did that, they would find major problems with the Act.

Among his concerns is the fact that the law puts doctors in a difficult position. "It really opposes a number of theological beliefs [that are] core to Christianity, including one of the Ten Commandments, 'Thou shalt not kill'. That command has been a guiding precept of every culture deriving from a Judeo-Christian background for thousands of years. Modern society still takes a high view of it."

Even if no malice is intended, a good motive has never been a relevant consideration in assigning responsibility for a deliberate act that is otherwise criminal, he says. By handing over this right to a doctor it will create distrust from their patients, something that at times is already faltering. "I still get calls from people 24 years after I've retired for my advice surrounding concerns over advice given by their doctor. People need to be able to relate to doctors, not be afraid of them."

Even if no malice is intended, a good motive has never been a relevant consideration in assigning responsibility for a deliberate act that is otherwise criminal, he says.

Assisted dying also directly opposes a core belief that life is sacred and has value because God created it, David says. "A human life—from its beginning in utero to its natural end—is to be deeply respected, as we are all created in the image of God. Jesus never taught death was preferable to life; like it says in the Bible, he came to 'give life, and life abundant'. Death is antithetical to the purposes of God.

"After Jesus went to heaven, part of the disciplines' ministry, and the church's, was healing. We read about it in the first of the New Testament passages. They didn't practise killing people; they healed the sick. Healing is listed in the books of Corinthians and Romans as one of the gifts of the Spirit. Causing death is not listed there."

David says Christians are compelled to care for the sick, as many Bible scriptures and parables command it. "The parable of the Good Samaritan condemns those who speak about compassion but are not prepared to sacrifice the time and personal attention demanded for the solace of suffering people. It is one thing to promote euthanasia as a compassionate response, and quite another to make the sacrifices involved in bringing love, comfort and care to the dying. Euthanasia is a cheap, quick, secular way of handling an emotionally-fraught situation."

"The parable of the Good Samaritan condemns those who speak about compassion but are not prepared to sacrifice the time and personal attention demanded for the solace of suffering people. It is one thing to promote euthanasia as a compassionate response, and quite another to make the sacrifices involved in bringing love, comfort and care to the dying."

He says bearing one another's burdens includes supporting the most vulnerable members of society who will feel the greatest pressure to request assisted dying.

Yet while we are to attempt to relieve each other's suffering, it can be difficult because suffering is in the eye of the beholder. "Most people would be glad not to suffer but the question then is, do you kill those people to relieve their suffering? You can't measure suffering. There's no scale—just somebody's word for it. The doctors have no option but to accept the patient's definition and act on it. It takes the decision out of the combined hand of doctor, patient and relatives, and makes it solely the prerogative of the patient to determine what is sufferable and what's not."

I ask David why he thinks it's important others are involved in decision-making for very sick patients.

"We quite rightly say there needs to be informed consent of the patient. That person should make an independent, informed decision. But what it means is the doctor tells the patient the options and likelihood of recovery, and the patient is then expected to choose. Very few people are able to do that themselves. Very often they ask the doctor, 'What do you think is best?'. The doctor then consults relatives and talks it through with the patient. There should always be group decision-making in these things so the patient's best interest can be met."

David says not every doctor or nurse is good at providing information in a way people can understand. And even if they are good at it, the person facing death or a major operation finds it incredibly hard to make a decision.

David says not every doctor or nurse is good at providing information in a way people can understand. And even if they are good at it, the person facing death or a major operation finds it incredibly hard to make a decision. "Advocates for euthanasia claim that 'because God has given us free will we should be able to exercise it in relation to our death'. But society cannot function effectively if everyone is exercising their 'rights' regardless of others. Just as Jesus gave up the glory he had with the father, individuals must agree to forgo certain matters of self-interest.

"This viewpoint is counter to the prevailing liberal philosophy that glorifies individual autonomy as the ultimate ethical principle. Liberal autonomy leads people to demand the right to have themselves killed at the time and place, and using the methods they determine. It is, they say, 'a private matter and no one should interfere'. But it is not private: someone else must play a part in events. Euthanasia is a public act."

And David says it is a dangerous one. "The system will eventually develop into one where people will have it done without consent."

He is referring to cases in the Netherlands and Belgium where people can give advance directives, so doctors and family members can determine when assisted dying should be conducted, and the person is not required to consent at the time of the injection.

"David Seymour is right in one sense. In other jurisdictions which have introduced assisted dying… at the start there was nothing to fear with safeguards and eligibility criteria holding. But over time they have changed."

Gradually safeguards are eroded away by the very people who advocated for them in the first place, David says. "Those who set the system up will have disappeared. The next generation won't have been through the whole process we are going through; they won't have heard the arguments against it. They will just accept it as part of the way the health system is run. And they will change it. That's when things get into big trouble."

> **"The next generation won't have been through the whole process we are going through; they won't have heard the arguments against it. They will just accept it as part of the way the health system is run. And they will change it."**

While originally it was introduced to stop the suffering of a very, very small portion of people who are dying, over time it has become an almost social panacea, he says. "You can just about get it for anything at all. The chairman of the Belgium review committee says he thinks anyone who is suffering should have access to it. He's euthanased all sorts of people, even psychiatric patients who were at one time an absolute no-no."

One thing that particularly upsets David about the proposed law is there is no plan to help those who apply for assisted dying and are denied. He's got a point; internationally around a third of applicants are turned down for assisted dying because they don't meet the criteria.

"If a person applies and gets rejected, there is no attempt to salvage that person. All the legislation says is the person has to be told. There's no follow-up. There's no attempt to throw resources behind that person and help them with the state of mind they are in. They have nowhere to turn if they get that 'negative' result."

One thing that particularly upsets David about the proposed law is there is no plan to help those who apply for assisted dying and are denied. He's got a point; internationally around a third of applicants are turned down for assisted dying because they don't meet the criteria.

It's something that will surely propel people to commit suicide and is not meeting the duty of care, David says. The right response, particularly for Christians, is to provide companionship and practical help to the sick, lonely and disabled people in the community.

According to David, Christians should be prepared to allow God to determine the manner and time of their end, just as he determines their beginning.

"By his courage in facing his forthcoming death, Jesus gives us courage to face ours. Jesus trusted his father to see him through the most awful death experience. In such circumstances we experience God's closeness, comfort and strength in a special measure."

CHAPTER 23:

MUSTAFA FAROUK QSM

It's been a big week for the Federation of Islamic Associations New Zealand in the lead-up to the first anniversary of the Christchurch Mosque attack on 15 March. A memorial event was organised and then cancelled within 24 hours of its start time due to COVID-19 prevention measures. But federation president Mustafa Farouk is calm and relaxed as he answers his phone from his Hamilton home the day after the planned event.

The federation is an umbrella organisation for the around 60,000 Muslims living in New Zealand, and is broken up into seven regions.

Mustafa works as a senior food technologist at AgResearch, he's married with five children and moved to New Zealand 24 years ago. His Nigerian accent is still strong. "I come from a family of 14 brothers and sisters… Each African is responsible for three other people in their extended family. He will have some responsibilities to relatives... whatever is yours is for your whole family. It's a different way of doing life in my home country."

Mustafa first moved here with his wife and two young children after he landed a job, and intended to stay two years. "That tells you what I feel about the country. It is the best place to raise kids."

I want to know what impacts he thinks the EOLC Act would have on both Muslims and immigrants.

"For us, in everything we are supposed to do as Muslims, we try and keep people alive. In the Qur'an it says if anyone takes the life of any individual without any due legal process it is as if that person has taken the life of all humanity. It is very grievous. And we are not allowed to take our own life. The punishment for the person who does that is he will dwell in hell forever. We are talking about people who are in full control of their capacity. They know what they are doing."

"For us, in everything we are supposed to do as Muslims, we try and keep people alive. In the Qur'an it says if anyone takes the life of any individual without any due legal process it is as if that person has taken the life of all humanity. It is very grievous."

I haven't spoken to anyone yet who lays it out so black and white.

"That means anyone who is a Muslim will not assist a person to take their life. If they are told by the law to do that, then they are forced to do something that completely contravenes their own belief. It's very clear. That's from a spiritual point of view. It's very clear in the Qur'an."

Wanting to get a precise definition, I ask: What exactly is the Qur'an?

"The Qur'an is the word of God. He is our primary source of law. No one can change what is part of the Qur'an. No individual, living or ever, will have that power to change what is written. People have a choice to follow or not, but no one in their own religion or culture can sit down and say these verses should be changed.

"Our second primary source is the prophet Muhammad. He has made it very clear to not take the lives of innocent people or take our own life. The Qur'an was given to him [Muhammad]—and he was the one who demonstrated what the teachings meant."

To be honest, from a straight religious perspective, I grasp at what else to ask. From a Muslim perspective there's no exception or wriggle room. What about how it may influence immigrants within his community of believers?

"We have a lot of immigrants in our community and we believe many will be made vulnerable under the Act. People who are not 'well to do'. There are many who could consider themselves as burdens to their families; they are at times not in a place to make a good decision. They may opt to make their decisions to relieve their family.

"While many in our community are taught this [assisted dying] is wrong, they are also told to obey the law of the country they live in. Most of our community immigrated from countries where authorities are hardly questioned. We are worried they are more likely to be pressured by authoritative figures. If this becomes legal, it will erode our cultural and spiritual identity; there will be a separation between a culture and the law of the land.

"No matter how people discuss this, suicide is suicide. It becomes a justification and normalised. It may not happen immediately, but over time. There are things that were not normal in the past that are now. Why open the door?"

Mustafa struggles to understand why we are not spending our energy finding relief for people. "We are looking at a section of the community and saying these people are worthless. It's just finding an easy way out, instead

"We have a lot of immigrants in our community and we believe many will be made vulnerable under the Act. People who are not 'well to do'. There are many who could consider themselves as burdens to their families; they are at times not in a place to make a good decision."

of trying to help them be more comfortable or cure whatever their ailment is. I don't see this as a solution to any problem but is a problem in itself… If a person is in pain I should ask, 'How can I relieve them?' If they feel unwanted, 'How can I make them feel wanted?'. Just eliminating them is not the answer."

"We are looking at a section of the community and saying these people are worthless. It's just finding an easy way out, instead of trying to help them be more comfortable or cure whatever their ailment is. I don't see this as a solution to any problem but is a problem in itself…"

What would he suggest as an alternative?

"If you choose to die, stop taking the medication; don't ask someone else to do it. If you think you're capable, there's nobody who can force you to do that. This is about putting it on someone else. It's drawing other people into something that is not good.

"These people, if they are in full control of their capacity, have their right to say not [to] eat or drink. Like some who fast and deliberately protest. I would not encourage that, but at least that person has done it themselves. Why would you draw society into what you want to do?"

Where's the dignity in that, though? "There is no dignity to any assisted deaths."

Mustafa has a friend who has been told three times by doctors that he has a week or two to live. "And he has lived 13 years. I remember he said to the doctor, 'Are you God?' I'm not saying doctors have no knowledge or statistics, but they are still not God."

Would any religion consider assisted dying moral?

"I would like to see one belief system that says it's OK to knock off a person. The responsibility of everyone considered a shepherd in our community is firstly to protect the lives of who he's responsible for, and secondly to protect the property and honour of those people.

"There will be no religion that would say forget about a person's life. These laws will have no religious backing. Here we are spending a lot of money telling people not to commit suicide, we are bending over backwards to not discuss suicide publicly so young people won't kill themselves... and yet we are telling other people who are diseased that their lives are worthless. I'm not trying to be insensitive to people in pain; I'm saying we should work to find a solution. If everybody who was in pain was eliminated, why put in any effort?"

Is the connection between family members stronger for Muslims? How would it affect them if a family member decided to use euthanasia?

"A lot of Muslims come from cultures where extended family has a strong connection. If you decide you are going to take your life, there will be a lot of people who will not be happy with this wish. You will leave a lot of people sad. Imagine if a sibling has been trying to help their brother have a good life here, they have worked hard every day to support them, and then they decide to do the one thing that would mean they are going to hell… It would be very sad.

"Everybody is passionate about what they feel around this issue. But for me, for someone who is a strong believer, I believe it's not my own opinion that matters. It's easy for me because I'm a Muslim and religion is very clear. But even if I don't have a religious belief, I would rather work hard towards trying to keep people alive.

"This Act is not a step forward."

At times all this talk of the difficulty surrounding dying gets too deep and heavy. I'm grateful I get moments to relieve the intensity by reflecting on everything while sitting on my Swiss ball in my home office. With the door open I can look out at the native bush next door. Good coffee (and chocolate) also helps.

Many of us are turned off by difficult conversations in life, and many times in the interviewing process I have had to switch gears and think about lighter things. Have a good laugh. Or watch something humorous. I think we all regularly have to do that: find a way to unload so we can carry on.

I'm grateful for my children who override pensive moments with their demands for the toilet, or a drink. Or worse still, discovering the nappy rash cream. They interrupt my thoughts. They have no respect for autonomy. And it is helpful. True to form, my son is running down the drive at top speed, with glee in his eyes pronouncing "dinner is ready".

CONCLUSION

COVID-19 level-four lockdown has lifted and we emerge as a different nation. A transformation has occurred, some elements good and some bad. We will need to recover from the sacrifice it cost us to isolate, and create a new normal as we let go of what we have lost.

It has also provided us with an opportunity. An opportunity to change. To address things we may have been running from, or fighting against. To confront issues we have ignored. Now is the time. It's uncanny how parallel the nation's hibernating has been with this journey into the issues surrounding assisted dying.

As I emerge from the depths of my home office and close my laptop for the last time, there is a difference in me. Yes, I am looking forward to my favourite takeaway again, but I also feel a newness. Of clarity and conviction. Of sharpening.

The people I've met really have been the treasure in this hunt. I've appreciated people who have allowed themselves to be exposed and real. Their quality and intelligence, passion and kindness. Their sincerity. I hope it has been translated in the pages written. Among them is a unity in the desire and hope to remove suffering. And common threads of fear, sadness and grief that bind us.

I've discovered so many things I knew nothing about. And have been introduced to communities of people that I didn't know existed. People who have dedicated their lives to caring in secret. People who have overcome things that would overcome me. People who make the most out of life and what they have. They've let go of so much in order to appreciate what they get to keep.

So many have seen so much. They have experienced death and pain, and stood by people through it. Some have spent too long talking about it all; they struggle to face it anymore and acknowledge the emotional drain. Many have put their name and reputation on the line to speak out, on one side of this argument or the other.

Regardless of the result that comes, I know we have incredible people in our midst.

It's been a privilege to explore the realms connected with assisted dying and there have been a number of great challenges along the road.

One is the reality that the simplicity of what is being served is not as it seems. If assisted dying really was an easy decision we would not be voting in a binding referendum. The EOLC Act would not have taken years to get to where it is now. The Select Committee would not have received close to 40,000 submissions. Internationally, equivalent laws would be swiftly introduced with no qualms, rather than being rejected by the majority. If this really was the best solution to suffering, then doctors, ethicists, lawyers, religious leaders, and vulnerable people groups wouldn't be standing in the way; they would be lighting the way—or at least they would be out of the way.

But here we are.

Another difficulty faced is the reality that suffering at the end-of-life is happening. Death isn't easy. We all face a level of fear over the uncertainty of what's before us. Some take peace in their religious beliefs, others are confident in the care they will receive from those around them, but for many it is a daunting future. It's hard to find the 'positive take-aways' from death.

It's in this context the issue of assisted dying and the EOLC Act promises to bring security and relief. I have been disturbed at the thought that control over death can bring peace. Presenting death as a form of relief is tragic—especially if it's done prematurely, before all other forms of relief are considered. I believe this is what the EOLC Act actually does.

There's no guarantee a person is receiving the best care. Sure, they will get information about options, but there's no requirement their suffering will be fully explored and all attempts will be made to help. And while safeguards promise to protect from pressure and depression, there is evidence from overseas that they haven't always done that.

For some, this will be their only option. That, to me, is failure.

The risk is too high and the reward too small. That isn't good maths. Or morals. I'm grateful that we already have options available in palliative care that can bring relief to the extreme cases.

Suffering is far more complex than it seems. It can encompass a vast range of struggles. And so the solutions need to match its reach. There isn't one easy answer because it isn't one easy problem.

Will assisted dying be an answer to the very few? I acknowledge, I don't know. But even if it is, how will we find those few? How do we measure a justifiable case? And at what cost? The lives of many others are being risked for only the possibility of relief for a few. The risk is too high and the reward too small. That isn't good maths. Or morals. I'm grateful that we already have options available in palliative care that can bring relief to the extreme cases.

It's been interesting observing the discussion around autonomy and the EOLC Act. Comments from one of the originators of assisted dying still rings in my head: Philip Nitschke's statement that true autonomy can only be found when you have a drug in your cupboard ready to take whenever you want to. And that drug you must find yourself, you don't need a prescription. It highlights to me that true autonomy has to provide the ability for you to receive what you request, with no restrictions. And with no impact on your surroundings.

The EOLC Act does not provide this. Firstly, your ability to gain what you want is entirely checked by other people. You must get 'permission' from two doctors, and approval from a registrar and an oversight group. Secondly, you must meet eligibility criteria formed by the Government. Many people will be ruled out by this process. If your argument is entirely hinged on assisted dying giving autonomy, it is flawed. Personally I'm grateful for the 'flaws'—they are the only things standing in the way of this law being abused, however flimsy they are.

Autonomy to this level shouldn't be desired. Surely we aren't pig-headed enough to think we always make good decisions, all the time. That's why we have law, and don't live in an anarchy. We need to be cautious of this extreme autonomy that seeks to carve out 'self' from 'others'. It can deny the beauty of love that binds us together. One of the most meaningful connections in life is the impact we have on our world and on those around us. We shouldn't be controlled by others, but to deny our attachment is to sever part of our purpose.

I believe the argument for autonomy in the case of assisted dying is driven by something deeper. We need to address our fears of the future—whether it be by educating ourselves, by pursuing counselling to get loose from the trauma attached to observation, by making advance healthcare plans, or by getting better acquainted with death's reality. These all need to be done. Maybe if we stop running from issues surrounding death now, while we are strong and healthy, when it comes we won't be so afraid. And ill-prepared.

In facing all these fears I am reminded that we are looking at the difficult cases; we also need to be reminded of the many, many good stories. Fear can blow things out of proportion. It feeds on the potential of the negative. Hope feeds on the potential of the positive.

One element that has become a personal gripe along the way

has been the claim that dignity is wrapped up in independence. The glorification of DIY has degraded the sense of community. It's as though needing each other has become a weakness.

Look, in all honesty I squirm at thinking about wiping an adult's bum. But that isn't because of the adult: that's my own problem with faeces. And that problem has greatly been overcome with the introduction of babies. There is no connection between dignity and doo-doo. So we need to stop writhing about it. Dignity is what someone has purely because they are a person. A person's value is not defined by their function. Some of the most beautiful pieces of art in the world don't 'do' anything, yet they are worth millions. And that's just some paint on a piece of paper.

Fear can blow things out of proportion. It feeds on the potential of the negative. Hope feeds on the potential of the positive.

Another term being flaunted in this arena is compassion. Assisted dying has attempted to wear the couture of compassion since it's inception. It's close relative 'mercy killing' is already a familiar term to most. And like dignity, I believe it's interpretation has been contorted. The sense of feeling empathy for others should not drive us to the same position of despair they are in. Trying to find a solution while in despair is unhelpful. In fact, compassion is not found in the relief itself, but is the act of coming alongside and lightening the burden by being bound shoulder-to-shoulder with the person in the process.

You can be entirely compassionate, with or without agreeing to assisted dying. So let's separate those two issues. It's false to claim assisted dying is the only compassionate option for some. It's a misuse of the term completely in an attempt to manipulate someone into agreement.

It's got to stop.

You can be entirely compassionate, with or without agreeing to assisted dying. So let's separate those two issues. It's false to claim assisted dying is the only compassionate option for some. It's a misuse of the term completely in an attempt to manipulate someone into agreement.

Ultimately, to vote in the upcoming binding referendum we have to put aside our thoughts on the concept of assisted dying and look at the law that is lying in wait. Does the law protect? Does the law shift? Does the law sift?

The law must protect against coercion. But the onus really falls on two doctors to do their best in locating something that is, by nature, sly. And it's something most doctors don't want anything to do with. Coercion is often hidden underground and most of us may find it hard to believe it could even be present. But lawyers are often the ones wrestling with the subtle complexity of it in courtrooms. Cases of coercion put them in business. So it's of note that lawyers are among those saying the detection mechanisms in this law are too weak.

Good accountability can discourage malpractice, flush out law-breakers, and punish wrongdoers. But no doctors have been prosecuted anywhere in the world for breaking assisted dying laws. Why?

Cases have been tried in court, and even review committee reports acknowledge laws have been broken. But no penalties have followed. There is an agreement in all jurisdictions that there have been a number of unreported cases of assisted dying, despite laws requiring it.

In some countries the interpretation of loose definitions in the law are being written by review committees which carry no guarantee of impartiality. In other cases the courtrooms are prescribing meaning.

Our policy making processes in New Zealand mean amendments to our law will have to be worked through Parliament. The pro-euthanasia lobby group says this should provide security as no other nation has changed its law.

This was true until 2020. This year, Canada is in the process of approving a new bill as this book goes to print. It must include the removal of the eligibility criteria "death in the foreseeable future". The Netherlands has a bill from a minor party that was due to be presented to parliament pre-COVID-19. It is lurking in the dormitories waiting for lockdown to wrap up.

Americans using the lethal drug aren't doing it for reasons of pain but because of the loss of autonomy, or at least the fear of the loss. Studies show people don't want to be a burden. The loss of the simple pleasures in life has become life-threatening. Motivational factors are not what they seem to be. Is this the suffering we were attempting to relieve?

I don't believe those in support of assisted dying have evil intentions. But I believe their hope has been misplaced.

My concern is that this law will just sustain our insatiable pace of life, instead of it causing us to hit the pause button like COVID-19 is doing for us. Instead of giving an opportunity to re-evaluate what we do and why, it might tempt us to apply a quick-fix to a problem that requires a slower, more sustained shift in our culture. Death will once again be glossed over. Fear will be pandered to. And nothing great will be conquered as it should.

My charge is: don't be swayed by fear. Or convinced by the claim of autonomy. Or sold by its simplicity. Rather, let's solve the world's problems and heal the world's pain properly. A band-aid won't do.

I'm sorry so many have had such difficult times with loved ones at death's door. But can we come together and work through the trauma of those experiences? To heal so we can see clearly. To learn, and dismantle fear together.

Let our loved ones lead us to solutions—ones that are meaningful and truly human. We must refuse anything less.

I'm voting 'no' to the End of Life Choice Act. What will you do?

EPILOGUE

The End of Life Choice Act's goal of safely relieving suffering is a noble one. But sadly, I've found the proposed law misses its mark. Suffering is a multi faceted problem that infiltrates so many layers, and takes on too many forms. That suffering, when added to the mystery and fear of death, and the societal disconnection we have applied to it, creates one big, complex concoction.

This reality has put me in a predicament: I can't walk away from the journey by merely ruling out a failed solution—it feels too much like unfinished business. If the EOLC Act isn't going to deal with it, then there has to be a better way. And I believe there is.

Throughout my interviews and research, there have been many ingenious moments. Among them is a growing cluster of concepts that could collectively make an impact. Some powerful ideas have come directly from contributors; other answers were uncovered as motivational factors for hastened death were revealed. Standout themes emerged... And they're ones that can be applied immediately. Some can roll out over our country as a whole, while others will require an individual commitment.

I think their variation is a start to more appropriately and thoroughly meeting a very real need.

Palliative care needs to be improved

"I don't think it can be said that there is a problem with the state of our law... The law is not broken. The health system is. There are too many people... too many elderly, too many terminally ill, too many disabled people, whom the health system is failing.

"And if we are going to do anything, we should be pouring funds and resources into ensuring that those people get the care they deserve and need, rather than suddenly presenting this new solution of a quick-fix with a quick death." – **Richard McLeod**

Currently Hospice NZ is one of the primary providers of palliative care services in New Zealand. It cares for one in three Kiwis who die. That was 19,616 people in 2018, and the number is steadily climbing. The organisation receives just over 50 per cent of its funding from the Government—that's around $55 million annually. It has to find the other $45 million from private donors.

Could you imagine being rushed into the emergency department in a hospital and being told you would only receive help if you could fund half of the cost of your care? More funding from the Government needs to be allocated for end-of-life care.

Data produced by the Ministry of Health shows the number of people dying in the next 20 years is set to increase by 50 per cent. But students and junior doctors are receiving a woeful amount of relevant training. Medical students are not receiving a proportionate amount of attention in their curriculum—they only get a few days out of their five- or six-year programme with direct exposure to palliative medicine.

The number of doctors choosing to specialise in palliative care is also of concern. University of Auckland lecturer and palliative medicine consultant Dr Anne O'Callaghan says the shortage of palliative specialists means they are extremely busy and don't have time to teach students. This has resulted in a shortage of placements available. It's a self-destructive cycle. Health Workforce New Zealand has recognised palliative care as being probably the most vulnerable speciality at the moment.

We must find a way to inspire, honour and motivate more people to pursue this as their vocation of choice.

What are our options currently?

It's apparent most of us don't know what we can already choose when it comes to end-of-life care. There's confusion around what is already legal and possible.

Our existing options include refusing treatment or stopping it, refusing or turning off life support, or having a 'do not resuscitate' order. All of these options provide a way for a medical condition to end a person's life, 'letting nature take its course'. Sometimes a doctor would advise a course of treatment that will make a dying patient more comfortable but may also possibly shorten their life as a side effect. This is done with the intent to alleviate pain and suffering, not to kill.

Confronting death

Demystify death by empowering yourself with education. The mystery of the unknown can plague our imagination. We've got to take some of that power back by becoming reacquainted with the end of the road.

Learn about it. See it. Talk to people who deal with it.

The mystery of the unknown can plague our imagination. We've got to take some of that power back by becoming reacquainted with the end of the road.

I came across some very helpful resources in Hospice NZ's recent campaign #weneedtotalkaboutdying. Their website contains a number of ways to kick-start conversations, prompt personal processing, and to disintegrate some myths and fears. One particular clip called *What is it like to die?* talks through the process of dying, explaining natural responses your body will go through as it 'shuts down'. There are also helpful '5 ways' resources on topics like Ways to help someone who is grieving, Conversation starters for your family, and Ways to talk to your child about death. Fundamentals of Palliative Care learning packages are provided by local hospices. Consider signing up for one. Get equipped to deal with death.

Talk about your death with family. Obviously this is not the sort of topic you naturally banter about at the dinner table… but we do need to consider at what point it will become appropriate. Having to face the conversation in the light of a terminal prognosis is too late.

I can't help thinking it feels similar to considering when to write a will. It had never occurred to me until my husband and I signed up for a mortgage. Our lawyer offered to throw in a 'will-writing service' for free. That was a deal-sweetener. While the thought was bizarre to me at the time, on reflection it made good sense. Most of us hope our own death will make a gradual appearance in some far-off distant time. But that doesn't always happen. Why not choose a date on your calendar, clear out some time, and make it an evening discussion with family members?

I think some of us may have fears even talking about it with others. But don't save all the fear and anxiety until the moment of crisis. Be brave. Be prepared.

I think some of us may have fears even talking about it with others. But don't save all the fear and anxiety until the moment of crisis. Be brave. Be prepared. It may require working through the subsequent weeks as family members face questions and fears of their own. A third party may need to be called on to help. But like with all fear—on the other side is greater liberty.

Write an advance directive. Again, Hospice NZ has resources available to help. Consider things like your values and goals for care if you were to become seriously ill. Choose someone to speak for you if you were unable to speak for yourself. Find and fill in an advance directive form which can be found on the Hospice NZ's website. Get it signed in front of two witnesses and give a copy to your family members and doctor.

Read good books. Dr Ira Byock has been a name popping up in my research. He is a palliative care specialist, advocate and author. I read some of Ira's book *Dying Well* and was immediately engrossed. Ira took stories from patients' deaths, including that of his father, to tell stories of love and reconciliation in the face of tragedy. It was a healthy way to experience what dying looks like through someone else's example. Ira provides a medical perspective and an interpretation. Another book of his, *The Four Things That Matter Most*, is helpful also.

"There is a richness to this difficult time of life that the general culture doesn't know. I've been trying to put into the culture some illness narratives that emit the human potential for wellbeing alongside the sadness and symptoms and difficulties with illness and dying. I'm not trying to romanticise it. I'm just trying to take off the blinders we have in our culture to see that concomitant with the difficulties, there is also value possible," Ira says.

Pursue release from having watched loved ones die

Nearly all of us have had traumatic experiences with loved ones near death. But I think many of us have filed the experience in the back of the cabinet under the label of 'that's just life'. What we may not so easily recognise is that this file gets pulled out when we address any current or future decision-making around death. And we may be fighting its effects daily without even recognising its origin.

There are screeds of scientific research on trauma. But here are some relevant standouts I have found...

There is such a thing called 'fear-based trauma', and it is caused by a bad thing we experience or witness. It can include receiving a serious or terminal illness, or news that is so overwhelming or shocking we cannot cope.

There is also 'loss trauma'. It occurs when there is a sudden and unexpected death or loss of a loved one after a difficult, prolonged illness. It can happen when there has been a series of losses without time in between to recover. Or intense, prolonged or suppressed grief can cause it.

'Emotional trauma' can include overwhelming guilt, coined 'survivor's guilt'. It can happen when someone is forced to do something against their nature or will, having their 'no' taken away.

All three types of trauma, if left unresolved, can impact a person in different ways. There could be physical effects like changes in sleep patterns, loss of hair, unexplained aches and pains, effects on the immune system, dreams and nightmares, or a person could become easily startled.

Emotional indicators include fear and anxiety, panic attacks, hyper-vigilance, an inability to rest, depression, 'numbing' addictions, feelings of helplessness and being out of control, or a need to be in control.

Trauma can affect the conscious, unconscious and subconscious memories in the brain. Stress created by trauma elicit responses from the amygdala, hippocampus and prefrontal cortex.

Common ways people get stuck in trauma is by minimising, justifying, defending, blaming, avoiding or forgetting in an attempt to avoid the effect.

These responses sound familiar to me. I wouldn't be surprised if all of us are carrying a degree of trauma. We need to get help. Find a counsellor who specialises in trauma. If you're religious, get prayer. Pursue ways to remove trauma from your life.

Better serve those with terminal or chronic illnesses

Be a friend. Be present. Vicki Walsh provided some insight into this. My last question to Vicki was, 'How do we help support someone who has terminal illness?'

Vicki told me a story of a close friend who struggled after hearing about Vicki's terminal diagnosis. The friend didn't know how to handle the news and totally disconnected from her. "Several months later the friend came back asking to meet up. She was standing there with flowers and burst into tears. She said sorry. Now we message each other every day, even if it's just a 'kiss' on messenger."

Vicki says a big part of their friendship was going for runs together, and once she had got sick they could never do that again. Since then, her friend has pushed Vicki in a wheelchair through three marathons. "We've found a way to run again together even though we can't. Be that kind of friend to someone—one who finds a new way to be together."

Be a hope-maker

A profound revelation Professor Margaret Somerville introduced me to was the understanding that hope is grounded in a sense of connection to the future, and that we can actually produce it. Hope is not a feeling. We are not a victim to it. It is not passive. Even if someone doesn't have a long-term future, it doesn't disqualify the value of short-term experiences.

"Hope involves a sense of connection to the future, a feeling that what we do now will matter in the future. It makes us feel that we will be part of the future. Without hope our human spirit dies; with it we can overcome even seemingly insurmountable obstacles," Margo says. We can help create and provide these meaningful moments in someone's calendar. We can 'make' hope.

Margo referred to a statement made by Viktor Frankl, a prominent Jewish psychiatrist and neurologist in Vienna who was arrested and transported to a Nazi concentration camp with his wife and parents. Three years later, when his camp was liberated, most of his family, including his pregnant wife, had perished—but he, prisoner number 119104, had lived. His story is staggering.

In *Man's Search for Meaning*, which he wrote in nine days about his experiences in the camps, Viktor concluded that the difference between those who had lived and those who had died came down to one thing: meaning.

As he saw in the camps, those who found meaning even in the most horrendous circumstances were far more resilient to suffering than those who did not. "Everything can be taken from a man but one thing… the last of the human freedoms—to choose one's attitude in any given set of circumstances, to choose one's own way."

"Everything can be taken from a man but one thing… the last of the human freedoms— to choose one's attitude in any given set of circumstances, to choose one's own way," says Nazi concentration camp survivor Viktor Frankl.

Viktor worked as a therapist in the camps, and in his book, he gives the example of two suicidal inmates he encountered there. Like many others in the camps, these two men were hopeless and thought that there was nothing more to expect from life, nothing to live for. "In both cases, it was a question of getting them to realise that life was still expecting something from them; something in the future was expected of them."

For one man, it was his young child, who was then living in a foreign country, Viktor says. For the other, a scientist, it was a series of books that he needed to finish. "When the impossibility of replacing a person is realised, it allows the responsibility which a man has for his existence and its continuance to appear in all its magnitude.

A man who becomes conscious of the responsibility he bears toward a human being who affectionately waits for him, or to an unfinished work, will never be able to throw away his life. He knows the 'why' for his existence, and will be able to bear almost any 'how'."

Where do we start? Why not schedule regular visits to extended family if you don't already, particularly ones who may be sick or possibly a bit lonely. Chat to the widow on the corner down the road who spends hours meticulously trimming her hedges and watering her flowers. If you have children, no matter their age, think about making it a family tradition to visit a rest home with flowers for residents once a term. Start small. It may surprise you how big the effect will be.

These are just some of the ways we can improve the process of dying, to support those suffering, and overcome our fears. There will be many more yet to be discovered.

I invite you to join the conversation and share your ideas on this books' Facebook page at fb.com/TheFinalChoiceBook

---

A GOOD ENDING

One afternoon while researching the effect of observational trauma on family members of a loved one dying, I came across an interesting person: palliative care clinical specialist and psychiatrist Associate Professor Sandy McLeod.

Sandy works at Christchurch and Burwood hospitals, and as a Hospice NZ clinical advisor. He was called on by the Attorney-General to provide an affidavit for Lecretia Seales' case before the High Court.

Funny enough, Sandy McLeod is no relation to Richard McLeod, or Roderick MacLeod. It's all mere coincidence I've interviewed the three with links back to the common Scottish clan whose motto is "hold fast".

Sandy's affidavit presented in court considered a number of issues in relation to psychiatry and assisted dying, but also included his prediction on Lecretia's final moments of life: it would be quick. I was lucky enough to catch Sandy by phone to ask him about it.

Sandy said he knew Lecretia professionally before she got the brain tumour, which added poignancy to the issue. "Lecretia was fearful about how she would die, and that she would lose her competency, and her brain. But based on her case I was given to review, I found her fears of a terrible death, as she described it, were unlikely," Sandy said. "And events proved me right."

Lecretia's fears were not realised. Her story ended well. That's the conclusion we wish for all.

FURTHER RESOURCES

Hospice NZ:

#weneedtotalkaboutdeath campaign including a clip called *What is it like to die?* found under the 'Hospice Care' tab at hospice.org.nz

Canadian Virtual Hospice:

Search *Final hours at the bedside: Is my loved one suffering?* online to find a useful video from the Canadian Virtual Hospice. A number of other videos produced by the hospice can be found on virtualhospice.ca

Local documentaries about assisted dying:

TVNZ1 Sunday Documentary, search *Live and Let Live TVNZ* at YouTube.com

International documentaries about assisted dying:

BBC documentary, search *Euthanasia doctor: 'I don't call it killing'* BBC Stories at YouTube.com

Dateline documentary, search *Allow Me To Die: Euthanasia in Belgium* at YouTube.com

Books:

Dying Well by Dr Ira Byock

With the End in Mind: Dying, Death and Wisdom in an Age of Denial by Kathryn Mannix

Where to get help 24/7:
Worried about your or someone else's mental health?

In an emergency
Call 111

New Zealand Suicide Helpline
0508 828 865

Need to talk?
Call or txt 1737 for the National Telehealth Service mental health and addiction helpline

Lifeline
0800 543 354 or txt 4357 (HELP)

Youthline
0800 376 633

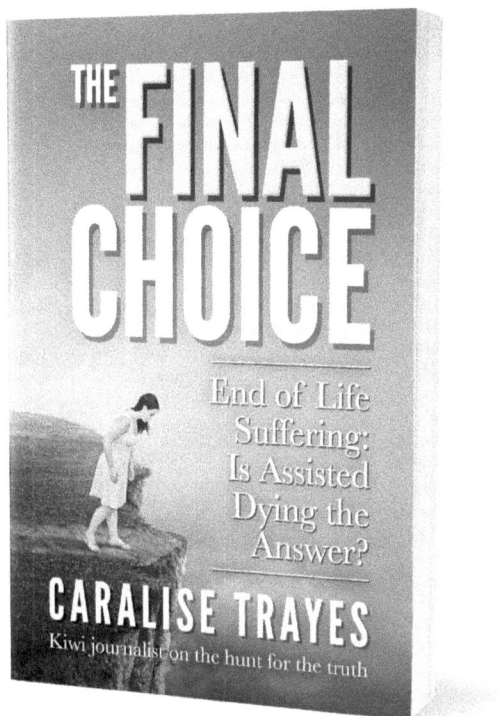

Join the conversation.

Like my page on Facebook at
www.fb.com/TheFinalChoiceBook

"I'd love to know your thoughts and hear from you. Engage in the discussion, share the page, and together let's make the best choice possible for our future."

Caralise Trayes

www.ingramcontent.com/pod-product-compliance
Lightning Source LLC
Chambersburg PA
CBHW071548210326
41597CB00019B/3166

* 9 7 8 0 4 7 3 5 2 4 5 1 7 *